Faster

The Obsession, Science and Luck
Behind the World's Fastest Cyclists

Michael Hutchinson

BLOOMSBURY
LONDON · NEW DELHI · NEW YORK · SYDNEY

BY THE SAME AUTHOR

The Hour: Sporting Immortality the Hard Way
Missing the Boat: Chasing a Childhood Sailing Dream

Bloomsbury Sport
An imprint of Bloomsbury Publishing Plc

50 Bedford Square   1385 Broadway
London   New York
WC1B 3DP   NY 10018
UK   USA

www.bloomsbury.com

BLOOMSBURY and the Diana logo are trademarks of
Bloomsbury Publishing Plc

First published 2014
This paperback edition published 2015

British Library Cataloguing-in-Publication Data
A catalogue record for this book is available from the British Library.

Library of Congress Cataloguing-in-Publication data has been applied for.

ISBN: PB: 978-1-4088-3777-1
        ePub: 978-1-4088-4374-1

2 4 6 8 10 9 7 5 3

Typeset in Bembo by Saxon Grahics Ltd, Derby
Printed and bound in Great Britain by CPI Group (UK) Ltd, Croydon CR0 4YY

MIX
Paper from
responsible sources
FSC® C020471

To find out more about our authors and books visit www.bloomsbury.com. Here
you will find extracts, author interviews, details of forthcoming events and the
option to sign up for our newsletters.

Contents

INTRODUCTION

An accidental athlete

WE ALL MAKE SACRIFICES TO FEED OUR PASSIONS. IN MY CASE, I can barely remember the last time I spent the night anywhere other than in a tent. This would be understandable were I a survivalist, a Bedouin or a terminally lost arctic-explorer, but I'm not. I'm a cyclist.

The tent is in my bedroom, which most people seem to feel makes things not quite as adventurous, but no less peculiar. I sleep in it because it simulates high altitude – the air inside has been pumped through a filtration system to reduce the oxygen content from the normal sea level 20.9% to something more like 14%. It's the equivalent of 3,500m, further up than Europe's highest mountain pass. Sleeping at 'altitude' this way is supposed to give you most of the benefits of altitude training without the inconvenience of living and working at the top of an Alp for 12 months of the year, or moving to Albuquerque.

That's not to say there are no downsides at all. The pump makes a noise like an outboard motor. On a warm night the temperature inside the tent can climb into the unbearable, and on a cold one the condensation drips down the inside until it saturates the sheets and I end up trying to sleep on a tiny sliver of dry in the middle of the bed. If I run a small fan inside the tent it can help with the heat and condensation problems, but then the noise of that combines with the outboard motor to replicate the effect of sleeping on an airliner.

The other inconvenience is my partner. Her first introduction to the tent was when she got home from work one night to find it already fully installed. I hadn't had the nerve to mention it. I suppose I hoped the surprise of finding it would distract her from the surprise of how much money had vanished from our bank account to pay for it. Since we lived in a one-bedroom flat she was either going to have to share it, sleep on the sofa, or just cut her losses and get out of the whole relationship.

I didn't show her the bit of the instruction manual that promised suffocation to those who attempted to share the limited air supply. The way I saw it, the less air there was to go around, the higher the effective altitude, and at no extra cost. I was untroubled by how closely this was related to the plastic-bag-over-the-head altitude-simulation system. This was simply because the tent was something that might help me ride a bike faster. I already trained more or less all day – now I could use those wasted hours of sleep to sneak another gain. I'd have bought the tent even if the warning was one of a random 30% chance of sudden death. Anything for speed.

I like to think that none of the foregoing would make anyone question my sanity. But even I have to admit that a rational man would have his doubts when I say that to this day I have no idea whether the tent and all its associated costs and aggravations actually made me any faster. The theory is sound, there have been a few reasonably good scientific studies, but even the best of those only claims it makes a relatively small difference, for some people, some-times. For me, perhaps multiplied by perhaps is enough.

It's not just the tent. In the same period I rode somewhere around 175,000 miles. I owned around 50 bikes, each one of which I was convinced was going to go faster than the previous one. I even spent a morning riding round Manchester Velodrome's track in the nude in an attempt to find out if bare skin was faster than a Lycra suit. (It wasn't, and thank God for that.)

I spent hours in laboratories being tested and measured. I'm an unusual physical specimen, so there was never any shortage of physiologists keen to poke and prod. I found out all manner of unlikely things about myself – I had what was reckoned to be just about the highest ratio of lung-capacity to height measured in a UK lab, for instance – that would have made interesting, if creepy, conversation starters at parties if I had not been so scared of catching a cold that I avoided parties at all costs, along with cinemas, and concerts. I sat on planes with a polo-neck jumper pulled up to just below my eyes, like Wilfrid from the *Bash Street Kids*.

I lived in a world where, one way or another, everything was divided into things that might make me faster and things that might make me slower. Pretty much anything pleasant fell into the second category. Eating sensibly makes you faster. A couple of beers make you slower. A quiet evening with your feet up to recover from a hard day on the bike makes you faster. A night out with your friends makes you slower. But misery and loneliness make you slower too. You don't have to be happy, and you almost certainly aren't, but you have to be able to function sufficiently to get up, have a kilo of porridge for breakfast, and get on your bike. Even the most committed have to choose between speed and sanity. So the question is: how much more committed will you be to next week's workload if you go out for a drink, and try to get riding right, eating right and thinking right out of your mind for an hour or two? Will you lose 3% of the week's progress, but gain 4%? Always running in the background is an app that asks, 'How do I go faster?'

I never meant for any of this to happen. I never even wanted to be an athlete. My ambition was to be an academic lawyer, and by my mid-twenties that's exactly what I was. I taught slightly left-wing civil liberties and human rights courses to first-year undergraduates at Sussex University. Since most of the students had their hearts set on becoming big-shot lawyers for major corporations, my job was overshadowed by the unspoken irony that my flock was almost certainly going to spend more time oppressing minorities than defending them.

I wasn't really too bothered by this, nor by knowing that they'd earn five times my salary while they did it. But I was driven to despair by the interminable Wednesday afternoon meetings of the faculty staff. Hours spent achieving nothing in an airless 1960s seminar room where the unjustified use of a gender-specific pronoun was fighting talk. We would debate such things as the political significance of the sign on the women's toilet featuring a figure standing legs-together, and the men's featuring one standing legs-apart. Or rather, older members of the faculty would debate it, while I and a couple of the younger members of staff would pass each other sarcastic notes about them under the table.

By then I'd been cycling for a couple of years, and I was getting quite good at it. I'd begun spending my weekends travelling up and down the UK to national-level races. I often abandoned work at lunchtime to do a few hours training, making up the time by working into the night. I resented every minute spent in the faculty meeting because it was a minute I wasn't on my bike. This quickly progressed to resenting every minute of my job because it was a minute I wasn't on my bike. My contract came up for renewal, and I don't think I even bothered going to the interview. Maybe it happened one Wednesday afternoon while I was down the corridor trying to work out which toilet to use.

I went to a research job at a different university. Or rather I took the money and the accommodation, and spent my time cycling. A successful season followed. A bike manufacturer offered me a contract to go full-time. The money wasn't great, and it would almost certainly be the ruin of my proper career,* but I said yes anyway. The obsession with faster had taken hold, and the chance to work at it undistracted by any more grown-up responsibilities was too much to resist. In some ways nothing I've done since in the pursuit of speed has been quite as irrational.

It led me into an odd career. I was a time-trial specialist, and I was in the only country in the world where you could conceivably make a living doing that. Unlike everywhere else, in the first few years of the twenty-first century the UK was still obsessed with time trialling as the bedrock of the sport. It suited me perfectly. Unlike mass-start road racing, TTing is an event for the analytical. It rewards hard work, knowledge and research. It's about control, in racing and training, about measuring efforts perfectly, and concentrating on what you're doing.

It's not mercurial. It's not especially interesting to watch, if I'm honest, at least not for a casual spectator. But it's the purest form of bike racing, and it finds the strongest riders. It's about speed, and nothing more. If you want to win a time trial, all you have to do is be the fastest rider in the race. There are no tactics, no teams, just you. From the inside it is fascinating, and it fascinated me.

* And it was so.

There was another reason I was happy with it. My career coincided with the dirtiest era in international pro cycling. That was where my background probably made a very serious difference to my riding. I didn't grow up as a star-struck kid dreaming of a life in cycling, or in any other sport. I bumbled into it almost by accident, and at an age where I was quickly under no illusions about how pro cycling worked. I didn't have hopes dashed, or agonising choices to make between my dreams and my honesty.

I knew what that world was like, and I wanted nothing to do with it. A friend of a friend went to Italy to try to carve out a career, and came back a few weeks later in despair. 'You can cheat or you can lose,' was his comment. 'Your choice.' Like a lot of honest riders of that era, I was a victim of the doping that was rampant. At the time I didn't really mind, because I had other options in life. I didn't feel trapped or disappointed. I just felt content to be scratching a living doing something I'd otherwise have been doing for nothing.

As time has passed I've come to resent it more. I can't help thinking that in a different time, or even a different sport, I could have been a star. Towards the end of my career I've become more competitive against the world's best riders than I ever was in my prime because the world's fastest bike riders are not quite as fast as once they were. The sport is finally making inroads against doping, and you can see it in the fact that since about 2006 the top pros have slowed down. Ten years ago, if I went to race a time trial against the very top riders I got beaten by margins that you could mark out on a calendar. In the last few seasons, it's down to a something you can measure in seconds, with perhaps even the occasional win.

I didn't really mind at the time, though, and I'm not sure there's a lot to be gained by minding now. I'm grateful that, for the moment at least, the sport has moved a long way in the right direction, and that young riders can find honest role models.

In my analytical little time-trial specialism I won more than 50 British titles over various distances, and as a dual-national I also won the Irish championships. I set numerous national records, including one that I took from Bradley Wiggins, was placed fourth at the Commonwealth Games on two occasions, and rode at the World Championships. I might not have reached the very top, but what I did I did clean, properly clean, and however self-congratulatory it might sound, I'm proud of that. I was, and I still am, a very fast bike rider.

The first question is: why? What is it about me that makes me faster than the vast majority of bike riders? Is it physical? Mental? Is it something innate, or something I achieved by training? There was a phase early in my career when I was so terrified that whatever it was might suddenly vanish that my first race of the year was a source of acute pre-event anxiety. Whatever it is was always there when I needed it, but that doesn't solve the mystery of where it came from in the first place.

The second question is: why are a lucky few faster than me? Is it just more of the same thing that makes me faster than everyone else?

The third question is: can I do anything to catch them?

These questions have had a hold over me for the last decade and a half – a large proportion of my adult life. It's no sensible preoccupation for a grown man, I know that. But I can't help it.

At least I'm not alone. Over the last few seasons I've had more and more people to keep me company in my obsession. For those of us interested in drug-free speed, the reduction in doping has had significant consequences. As one coach put it to me, 'Six or seven years ago, who the hell was going to look for a 1% gain from better training if they could inject a 10% gain with better drugs?' If you wanted to go faster, in a sport with a doping culture, pharmaceuticals were always going to be the most cost-effective place to spend your time and money.

One of the sport's more powerful players gave it a broader context: 'Ten years ago, a team's budget comprised one-third rider salaries, one-third logistics, and one-third drugs. The core skills were pharmacology, doctors, how to avoid detection, and how to move the whole operation around the world without getting caught. The teams were very good at this. But most of them had very little knowledge of genuine coaching and conditioning of riders. Then in the last few years, teams have had to get out of the systematic doping game. There's a third of the budget going spare. A lot of them spent it on rider salaries. But some of them spent it on coaching, equipment, sports science support.'

In short, there has never, in the whole chequered history of cycling, been more interest in non-pharmaceutical ways to make riders go faster than there has been in the last few years. Ten years ago a lot of clean amateurs had a more sophisticated grasp of training, aerodynamics and associated arts than the top pro teams did, because the top pro teams had better (for which read 'worse') things to worry about. In many ways, pro cycling has become much more like amateur cycling, or like the kind of thing I've been doing all my life.

The idea that the doping culture meant that every other aspect of cycling performance was underdeveloped is one that I found was supported by almost all the sports scientists and coaches that I talked to, from within cycling as well as without.

Sir Dave Brailsford, the boss at Team Sky, accepted that this backdrop was part of the reason for their success: 'In a sense it was a fluke, the sport was cleaning itself up just as we arrived, with a different skillset that we transferred from the national-squad track programme. We spent less on big-name riders, and more on full-time coaches, performance analysis, psychology, and sports science.'

It's not surprising that Team Sky would want to take as much from the Team GB approach as they could – the GB squad has been quite outrageously successful over the last few Olympic cycles. It's probably been the most successful sporting campaign in history. The sudden availability of lottery funding from the late 1990s onward was certainly the basis for it, but the money wasn't infinite, and it was spent efficiently.

The lottery cash was aimed at generating Olympic success, following a national panic after the 1996 Games when the British team came home with just a single gold medal. Since Steve Redgrave and Matthew Pinsent were such unsurprising winners the medal almost didn't count. Peter Keen, the first director of the new-look GB cycling team, concentrated exclusively on the events where he reckoned Olympic medals were easiest to win. That meant staying away from the road entirely – too many drugs, and tactics-dominated racing that was too unpredictable – and putting all the resources into track racing, which by the late 1990s was a backwater that no nation had invested in properly since the fall of the Iron Curtain.

It was more focused even than that – the investment went into the quantifiable, controllable events with the lowest possible risk. The 1km time trial, the team sprint, the individual pursuit and the team pursuit got the cash, because they were races of pure speed. Other events, like the match sprint and the points race, which depend on tactics and a bit of luck, were largely ignored. If it didn't generate a number for the spreadsheet, it didn't get done. It was a ruthless, lean system designed to turn money into medals.

I was, for a while, a handful of cells on the spreadsheet. I spent a couple of years not quite on, not quite off the track squad. To get properly on to the squad, I had to make a qualifying standard time of 4'30" over a 4,000m pursuit. It was obvious to the coaches that I had the capacity to do this, but, though I repeatedly got to within a few tenths of a second of it, I never quite made it. The head coach at the time tried manfully to get me the last few yards. He kept me around the programme longer than he probably should have done. But it never happened.

My problem was, ironically, that I was a professional rider on the road. My success there depended on judging a sustainable time trial effort over distances much longer than 4,000m, and I was too good at it. I struggled very badly to raise my pace above the effort levels that I knew so well, because every time I pushed properly into the red zone all my carefully trained alarm bells went off.

With hindsight, what I should have done was abandon the road career, give up that income, and focus on the track. If I'd done that, I'd have made the time, got myself on the squad, got the resulting funding, and more to the point, got access to the coaching and support that was available. I didn't. It was a huge mistake.

I got to watch a lot of people I'd ridden with, gone on training camps with, winning medals at the 2004 and 2008 Olympics. They had the opportunity to do that because they produced the results for the spreadsheet when it mattered. I knew that was how it worked when I got involved, so it was no one's fault but my own.

This is the sharp end of a team. The aim is for the team to win medals, not to help any given individual make the most of themselves. It's Darwinian. When I interviewed Shane Sutton, the head coach of the GB team for London 2012, he said simply, 'I'm trying to win medals, to get the funding, to make sure all these people have a bloody job next year.' He gestured round an office full of team staff. 'It's the system that has to win.'

The system lived by what became known as 'the aggregation of marginal gains'. It's a phrase that seems to mean different things to different people. I think the simplest understanding of it is that it's about looking for any way to go faster, however big, however small, and it works by breaking everything down into its component elements to see if you can make any improvement to any one of them. One comparison might be the script room of a major US sitcom. The writers don't look at a whole show and ask if it's funny enough, they take the script to bits, look at every scene and every single line, and no matter how funny it might already be, they ask whether there is any way to make it funnier, all the way down to the individual words.

So 'marginal gains' doesn't just look at diet, it looks at diet before training, during training and after training. Then before, during and after one-day races. Then how that regime would have to be altered to deal with the different demands of stage races and Grand Tours. It looks at how to serve up what's required in a way that makes it easy for an athlete to eat it. Ultimately it hires a chef, because that's the only way 'marginal gains' can solve all the problems of the right nutrients in the right food in the right place at the right time.

'Marginal gains' doesn't just exhort riders to have a good night's sleep – it examines the post-training and racing routines and commitments that affect bed-times, it researches the best earplugs, it buys eye-masks and MP3 files of rainforest sounds, and it packs each rider's pillows into the back of a van and drives them to the hotel.

'Marginal gains' doesn't give a toss what anyone else thinks. Team Sky decided that since the first step to good post-race recovery was a warm-down, they'd make sure that for races that finished with a flat-out effort, like a hill-top finish, the riders would get on to stationary trainers after they'd finished and warm down properly. The reaction from other teams was unrestrained mirth, at least for the two or three months it took for them to start doing the same thing.

It's not really the gains that are marginal – some will be small, but some will be big. It's where you go looking that's marginal, peering into every nook and cranny of cycling. In the run-in to 2012, the GB track team looked at plenty of things that ultimately turned out to be unimprovable, or at least not without creating considerable knock-on difficulties. Wheel nuts could be made more aerodynamic, for example, but only at the cost of being almost impossible for the mechanics to work with when the pressure was on.

You have to keep looking, all the time. Sport moves on. It gets better, it gets faster. If you stop to catch your breath, you go backwards. I always reckon I need to find about 2% a year from somewhere just to stay where I am in the pecking order. Until I find that 2% I'm not even making any real progress.

It's not a unique approach. One senior businessman working on a programme for the BBC went to British Cycling's base at Manchester Velodrome after the 2008 Games to see what lessons industry might learn from the team. He concluded that what was going on there wasn't very different from what the most successful businesses were already doing. But it was new to cycling, and it changed things.

Ultimately, I didn't ever make it to the very top of the sport. In an odd way, I'm grateful for that. It meant that I ended up focusing on the personal rewards of chasing excellence rather than on the financial ones, and I avoided the pressures that would have brought. There was always something to be said for being able to do more or less what I wanted. As I approach retirement, of course, I can't help feeling there might equally have been something to be said for the big house and the investment portfolio, but I try not to dwell on it.

My perch just below the summit of the mountain is a wonderful outlook if you want a perspective on the quest for faster. Chris Boardman pointed out to me during an interview that, 'At least you know what it's like.' He meant, generously, that I knew what it was like to compete at the top level, to have that all-consuming passion, to live a life governed by a stopwatch. But I also know what it's like to look up at the very best and wonder how they got there. I know how to win, and I know how to lose. If you don't learn more from losing than you do from winning, you're not doing it right.

This book was an excuse to write down all the things I've been worrying about for all these years. It was also an excuse to ask the best riders, coaches and sports scientists about what made the fast so damn fast. I learned a very great deal, and rather more than I expected. Partly this was because I knew less than I thought I did, and partly it was because in recent seasons things have moved on more and more quickly. I was surprised, and delighted, at the detail most of those I spoke to were prepared to go into about what they do. More than one rider said they were happy to tell me what they were doing, because just knowing what it was wasn't enough. You had to be able to *actually* do it.

Most people only see elite sport in its moments of glory. They never hear about the nether regions where the work gets done. Paul Manning, gold medallist in the team pursuit in Beijing, and coach of the women's endurance track squad at London, said that he reckoned at least 95% of the coaches' and riders' jobs had already been done before they even walked into the track for the first rounds of competition.

I'm not going to deal with the racing and the glory. I'm going to deal with the 95%, the basics of what makes an athlete. What it is about their physiology that allows them to do what they do, and how they came to be built that way. How they do their jobs, and deal with not just the pressures of competition, but how they motivate themselves when being a star consists of a wretched seven-hour ride through the freezing January drizzle. I'm going to look at the technical issues of aerodynamics that have become more and more prominent, and, finally I'm going to deal with the way genetics underpins all of human performance.

It's worth saying that this book is not intended to be a manual. It's not sufficiently comprehensive. There are certainly some things that the elite riders do that could be applied by anyone, but most of the book focuses on the small margins that separate the Olympic gold medallists and world champions from the athletes who were right behind them. To be blunt, for most riders it would be pointless to worry too much about the last tenth of performance gains until they've dealt with the first nine. As Olympic coach Dan Hunt said, 'It's a waste of time drinking organic cherry juice if you're using it to wash down a Big Mac.'

What the book does illustrate, I hope, is just what's possible when resources and ingenuity are brought to bear on the simple act of riding a bike.

CHAPTER 1

Like a racehorse: the art of being an athlete

ONE WINTER NIGHT, HEADING HOME AFTER MEETING SOME friends in a London pub, I caught the last train from King's Cross to Cambridgeshire. To avoid falling asleep and finishing up at the end of the line in King's Lynn, I took out some headphones and a notepad, and started to transcribe an interview with British pro Alex Dowsett.

Somewhere around Stevenage, I was concentrating on this when I saw a man in his early twenties coming over. He was already speaking when I took the headphones off. What he was saying finished with '...Alex Dowsett.' I'm confident the already slack jaw and the Sauvignon Blanc fumes managed to mask my confusion.

He'd been at school with Dowsett, and had recognised me as one of his friend's former opponents. He was an ex-international racer himself – when British Cycling's talent scouts had, in their best East German style, visited the school to check up on Dowsett, they'd picked him out of the crowd too. It had been a surprise. Cycling wasn't something he'd ever really thought about seriously.

'But they said they'd give me a decent bike, help me with training, enter me in a few races, and see how it went. I liked the idea,' he said. 'Who wouldn't?' He ended up racing as a junior at the World Mountain Bike Championships. He did well too, for a relative novice. The talent scouts had been right – he had what it took.

Or at any rate he had part of what it took. Why, I asked, had he given it up? It was simple, he said. He hadn't been an athlete. The excitement of racing hadn't made him want to spend months and years devoted to training. He'd been good at riding a bike, and that was all.

Dowsett, on the other hand, had been an athlete before the talent team even arrived. And while his friend and I pursued a slightly drunken (on my part anyway) conversation about bikes, books, and missed opportunities, somewhere in Essex he was sleeping the sleep of the going-to-get-up-in-the-morning-and-do-a-six-hour-training-ride.

There is a skill to being an athlete. It's not an easy job. You have to learn how to train. You have to learn how to work with a coach, and how to get the best out of whatever other support is available to you – something that quite possibly starts with finding that support in the first place. You have to manage a career, look after your body, and keep your motivation intact.

At what might seem like an absurdly basic level, you have to be able to tell when you're too tired. By any normal measure most athletes are very tired a lot of the time, and the edge that slips you into 'too tired' is almost imperceptible. 'Tired' isn't even a single feeling – fatigue comes in a hundred varieties, all of which you learn to analyse for signs of danger. Nor does it help that the whole idea of 'too tired' moves depending on where in the training cycle you are. What might count as just 'quite tired' six weeks before a major event would be 'much, much too tired' a week before.

Before the London Paralympics, Dame Sarah Storey used a block of training in an altitude chamber. This wasn't something she'd done before. 'I had to do it almost by ear,' she said. 'You put your face close to the mirror every day, and ask yourself how you feel, how you really feel. Good? Bad? OK? Is that a twinge? Or am I imagining it? But it's no different to usual. Training is never the same twice – what was fine one season might be too much the next. You always have to ask yourself how you feel. Always.'

Equally you have to know when things are good. Dowsett's first big pro win was the time trial stage at the end of the Tour of Britain in 2011: 'I'd written off the TT because the week had been so hard. But when I stood up out of bed in the morning I knew my legs were good. I knew the day would be OK, so come the race I made sure I got everything out.'

No one can teach you this ability to read your own body. It comes only with experience. A coach can help, they can ask questions, and they can try either to make you play safe, or perhaps push you to go a bit deeper if they think you should be able to cope, but they can't know how it feels from inside.

It's the same with training. You can have all the help in the world, but you have to do it yourself. I'd be the first to point out that having time to spend on something as trivial as training is a considerable luxury, but doing it well, doing it all the way to your limits, is a very tough way to spend your days. That's how it works. Paul Manning won gold at the Beijing Olympics, and coached the GB women's endurance squad in London. Referring to this squad, he said, 'Most people, most cyclists even, have absolutely no concept of how hard they train. Laura Trott is sick after some of the efforts – there are jokes about the bucket we take to training sessions for her. She'll push that hard again and again in one session. It's masochistic. She loves what she does but she comes to the track to ride hard.'

Chris Hoy used to do his static trainer sessions with a crash mat beside the bike, on to which he'd collapse in literal agony after an effort. Then he'd get up and repeat the process. This wasn't because he was in any way soft. It was because he was pushing himself to somewhere that only those who have practised doing it can ever reach. 'Back in the day,' he said, 'I used to do turbo trainer sessions. I'd set up in a stairwell at my parents' house, and I'd put myself through hell. Just on my own. No teammates for a bit of competition or anything. Just me. You can't rely on being inspired by anyone else. You have to want it yourself.'

It has to be hard. Time and time again I've asked star riders how they made the step up to the very top levels – I usually asked with a bit of an agenda because I felt as if it was the step they'd made and I hadn't. Almost always they said it was because somehow they'd found more within themselves with which to race and train. Often they were faced with a pro peloton that went faster than they'd believed possible. The speed of a race broke them through to a new place, a new 'hard' they never knew existed, but somewhere they could go back to on their own later.

Or maybe they grew up with a group of talented juniors, and they raised each other's expectations, work rates and tolerances: a group of teenagers who put themselves on the line again and again and moved their collective concept of the conventional on to higher and higher levels. The Isle of Man produced a group of outrageously good riders in the mid-to-late 2000s, including Mark Cavendish, and it wasn't a statistical anomaly.

The same thing can work on a broader scale. Sir Chris might have placed an emphasis on what you demand from yourself, but it's still hard to escape from the theory that part of the success of British Cycling over the last decade is the group of athletes training together at Manchester.

Watching each other, seeing what a rival for a place on the team can lift in the gym, constantly measuring up against each other, they create a bubble of their own extraordinary normality. It's a contrast to UK sports like athletics or swimming, where the athletes and their coaches are spread out over the country and only come together a few times a year. That's just competition, and that's not always enough.

I'm not sure how best to describe what the hard sessions are like. For a start, I'm not sure they feel the same for everyone, especially for sprinters when compared to endurance riders like me. I suspect that sprinters have to cope with more 'pain' (I'm not sure it's at all the right word – the sensations are positive, even if they're not enjoyable in the sense that most people would understand it) but that endurance riders have to do it more often. But I might be wrong. Nor am I even sure that my experience is representative of everyone else, even if their physiology is broadly comparable.

I know that the way I trained changed over my first few seasons in the sport. I don't mean the content of the sessions, I mean how I did them. I came to cycling from a different endurance sport (rowing), so I wasn't totally green when I started. I think what distinguishes a hard session done well from a hard session done badly is the degree of control. When you've grown good at it, you can push to the limits of what you can do while staying so relaxed that you can wiggle your toes. There's no trace of a wild attack on the effort. You can feel what you're doing, and judge the effort level, even while your heart rate is at its maximum and your blood-lactate levels are heading for the roof. There is a detachment. You're not just piling everything on and hoping for the best.

In the last couple of seasons my training has included a session of 'all-out' sprint efforts, over 30 seconds. The idea is to start as fast as you possibly can, to hit what would effectively be the biggest number you can hit under any circumstances, then just keep going as hard as you can manage so you're always hitting the biggest power number you're still capable of. The curve peaks after a couple of seconds, in my case at about 1,100 watts (or 1,100w), and then declines constantly for the rest of the 30 seconds until it gets to about 700w. Hence 'all-out' – it's not an evenly paced effort, it's about making sure you give everything you have. It sounds like a frenzy of effort, a spasm of sprinting. But when you do it well there is calmness and precision all the way through.

It's the same with other efforts – I do a 'pace-change' session of two minutes at 500w, a minute easy, a minute at 540w, a minute easy, and an all-out 30-second sprint. 500w for two minutes is the hard part of that – it's well above sustainable time trial pace. It's all I can do, and even then I can do a full set of repetitions only on my better days. But I'm still in control of what I'm doing. The 500w is 500w, it's not 490w or 510w. One of the Team Sky coaches said that their riders – especially those like Sir Bradley Wiggins with a track background – could do exactly the same. If a session calls for minutes alternating between 510w and 450w, they'll nail the numbers and the transitions right up to the point when they just physically can't do it any more. On the computer screen afterwards, the power curve looks like a battlement.

It helps, of course, that for elite riders the numbers haven't been produced at random – they're carefully worked out so that they're something very difficult but not impossible. Good coaches have a sense for where a rider's limits are. But hitting the numbers when the numbers are so demanding is a phenomenally skilful thing to be able to do, and it comes from years of practice.

That it 'hurts' is almost neither here nor there. You try to tolerate it, embrace it, put it in a box, luxuriate in it, turn your back and go to your happy place, deal with it in whatever other way you can. You have to go back again and again, and while you get better at it, it never gets easy. You need to listen to the sensations, because they tell you what's happening. But there are many times you need to do your best to just ignore it all, to go deeper, because that's part of learning how to train.

It's personal. Sports scientists have a scale of perceived exertion – named after the Swedish physiologist Gunnar Borg – that goes from six to 20: 11 is 'light'; 13 is 'somewhat hard'; 15 is 'hard'; 17 is 'very hard'; 19 is 'extremely hard' and 20 is 'maximal'.* I'm haunted in the night by the suspicion that what I think is a 20 is only a 15. Or that the people who are better than me got that way by the ability to hit 22, or 25 or 29. I once had some 'I've been to Borg 21' T-shirts made, but even the world of exercise physiology reckoned that was a joke too geeky.

I also worry that as I get older I've suffered from Borg inflation. I think that my ability to scale the heights of 19–20 improved as I learned to train, plateaued for several seasons, and is now in decline. I'm almost sure that my present-day 20 was only good for an 18 ten years ago. I've also developed a private suspicion that Gunnar Borg was just trying to make trouble inside the heads of people like me.

Training is not the only skill an athlete has to have. There are others that, even if they're not as physically unforgiving, are as important. You have to be able to take

---

* It starts at six because the idea was that the scale would be representative of the corresponding heart rate: six would be around 60bpm, ten around 100bpm, and so on. This is very approximate, and ultimately, in a modern world full of heart-rate monitors, not actually very helpful.

coaching, to absorb a lot of information about what you're doing, and act on it. In 2011 Tim Kerrison, the performance analyst at Team Sky, started to push the importance of riding a negative split in time trials – making the second half a little harder than the first. It might not be the absolute A1 fastest way to do it, but it's the safe way to get the whole effort out and the losses are minute compared to the benefits.

It's a little counter-intuitive for most riders. Some took this on board better than others – Wiggins was clearly putting it into practice at the Worlds that year and in the following season at the Tour and the Olympics. Dowsett (at that time a Sky rider) had always hit time trial efforts very hard from the beginning, and had more trouble with it. On one short prologue he hit a 470w average for the first half, and 410w in the second. He admitted that Kerrison wasn't massively impressed.

My own coach and I worked out a similar strategy on our own. We based it on computer-modelling courses and producing an optimised plan for riding them. Simple physics dictates that there is a benefit to be had from riding harder on the climbs when the aerodynamic drag is lower. (The power needed to overcome aerodynamic drag in a race increases as the cube of speed – getting where you're going twice as fast is eight times as hard. Gravity, on the other hand, is a simple geometric increase – twice as fast is only twice as hard. You get better value for your anguish by pushing on the hills.)

The differences are subtle. The model accounted for gradients, for weather, and for the individual physiology of the rider – some of us are better at recovering from excursions into the red zone than others. Even allowing for all that, the typical variation in pace is usually no more than a very subtle 10% above or below an average pace.

Despite the effort that went into the model, it's not really possible to ride a time trial course by just staring at the numbers on a little screen on your bars. The first problem is that some days your form is better than others, and a danger is that you pick the wrong numbers. Pitch too low and you give away time. Pitch too high and you end up trying to sustain an impossible pace, with inevitably disastrous consequences. The second problem is the near impossibility of memorising maybe 50 different course segments and their corresponding power requirement. The third problem is getting sufficiently accurate topographic data to feed into the model to begin with.

The art was in using the model as a guide, sitting down after a race with the computer file to compare it with the ideal to see where I got it right and where I got it wrong. I spent hours in front of a computer, relating the lines on the graph to the roads of the race, and the theory to the practice. I wanted to learn how to get it right just on feel. The differences are worth having – it depends very much on the details of the course and the physiology of the rider, but even on a relatively flat course you might find a second a kilometre just from laying down the right power in the right place.

This is the kind of thing with an inherent appeal only to the more nerdy end of the spectrum of riders. Most of them would rather just get on with riding their bikes. But anyone who is serious about riding a time trial has to work with the coaches and performance analysts and get used to it because it's a chance to go faster without having to find any extra physical grunt.

Sir Chris Hoy referred to this sort of thing as 'becoming a student of the sport'. You have to take it seriously, because the margins are so tight. Hoy's first world title, in 2002, was by one thousandth of a second – about 19mm over the course of a kilometre. He told me, 'You always want the best information, you want to talk to the best people. You can go to the wind tunnel, you can see exactly what distance you can gain if you keep your head down and your elbows in. Then you go and look at a picture of yourself in the final stages of a sprint with your elbows sticking out. It's not easy to change a style you've used for years, but you have to fix things like that. I watch videos of the best guys from the past, the 1980s, the 1970s – how did they do it? What tactics did they use? You can never be satisfied – even after the 2008 Olympics I went back to look for any way I could have gone any faster. You never get there.'

When it comes to details, the Hoy elbows are just the tip of the iceberg. Qualifying for a match sprint competition is a 200m flying-start time trial: 'You have to look at peak speed down to 0.1kph. Then you go back and look at where the optimal spot on the track is for the peak power, because every track is different. If your gear is too small, you'll hit peak power too soon, maybe even before reaching the 200m [start] line. When you get the gear right, then you have to apply the power in the right place – it might only vary by a couple of metres from one track to another, but you have to get it right. You need to know the temperature, the air pressure, because they matter too. You end up doing all this without really thinking about how subtle it is.'

When I was hanging around in Manchester in the early 2000s, busy failing to get on to the GB team pursuit squad, I spent quite a few nights in the squad house. It was the only still-occupied terrace in an otherwise boarded-up street behind the Velodrome, and was among the most frightening places I've ever been. If I'd been half as fast at the training sessions as I was at barrelling down the dark street afterwards, ramming the key into the lock, flinging myself through the door and locking it behind me I'd have had a much brighter track career than I did. If I was staying there on my own I used to wedge the sofa behind the door as well, and sleep with a heavy frying pan beside the bed. As feral teenagers howled like wolves in the street outside it was a comfort to remind myself that I was involved with one of the best-funded cycling teams in the world.

One night I shared it with a group of juniors, which included Mark Cavendish. It was the night of the Champions' League final. I put it on the TV. We all watched it for a few minutes, until one of the lads said, 'Do you mind if we watch something else? We're not really into football.' I'd found the only group of 17- and 18-year-old males in the country with no interest whatever in football.

What happened next was even more interesting. One of them produced several VHS tapes of races. He put one on, fast-forwarded to a sprint finish, and together they analysed the hell out of it. They scanned backwards and forwards for what felt like hours till they'd worked out exactly, and I mean *exactly*, why the winner had won and the losers had lost. 'What happened to Zabel?' 'He should have swapped to that Saeco guy's wheel there, cos his lead-out got hit by the crosswind there from that gap in the buildings.' 'Nah, if he'd done that, the Festina guy would have shoved him into the barriers. He's already in trouble cos he's stuck behind the Gan guy, and the Gan guy is in the wrong gear...' and so on, forever and ever. It wasn't the conversation a group of fans have, or even a group of journalists. It was much more serious, much more knowledgeable. They were revising for their next race.

These were riders who knew they had some talent, who wanted to succeed, and who knew what that meant. There was no danger whatever of them going to the local supermarket and bringing back a few tins of lager. There wasn't even any danger of them going to the local chip shop. They knew they'd got a golden opportunity, and they were not going to waste it.

That group of riders would be in their late twenties by now. When a more recent under-23 international told me about a training session that consisted of short sprint reps performed in an altitude chamber, I asked what the idea behind it was. He shrugged and said, 'I don't know. I don't have to know – I have people to know this stuff for me.' I was left wondering if there was a younger generation that was a bit less engaged.

When I made the suggestion to a number of coaches, though, for the most part they disagreed. Paul Manning said that the single biggest change since he'd been a rider was the level of knowledge that younger riders had, having grown up through a much more advanced sport, one where there was more information and help available than there was when he was coming through. He was adamant that even the younger riders in his squad were well able to lead their own programmes.

I'm not sure there is really all that much of a contradiction. For the old guard – Hoy, Manning, perhaps even Wiggins and, at a less-lavish pay-grade, me – the lack of sophistication in an old-fashioned-feeling sport enforced a degree of self-sufficiency. There simply wasn't the help available until you reached quite a high level, and until then you were probably on your own. Hoy's career was underpinned by a degree in applied sports science. I used to kill lunchtimes in the university library reading physiology journals. Even if I was usually holding the wrong end of half a dozen sticks at the same time, I was still better off than most.

Now the help is easier to find, and that has changed how riders develop. Dowsett said that he appreciated it as a 'knowledge base' that he could tap into. 'I've always had a team of some sort, British Cycling or a trade team, behind me so I haven't had to find things out on my own. I'm doing things that I know work. I have faith in them.' For that generation it's no longer a case of struggling to work things out for themselves, it's a case of taking on board what's there.

You could still ignore it all and just do what you're told. It's a lot more likely to work now than it was 20 years ago when the most readily available advice was either a magazine article or your mother. The former was hampered by its mandate to help everyone from the gifted 14-year-old to the middle-aged donkey without killing either, the latter by a perverse perception that your education ought to take priority over your bike riding.

In the end, the most successful riders seem to be those most closely involved in what they're doing. It means they can cope if things go wrong. It provides motivation. At its best, it's an attitude that goes beyond the day-to-day life of training. If you're a proper part of the process it makes what you're doing into a career rather than a job. It's telling that when Dame Sarah Storey switched sports from swimming to cycling, she made a conscious effort to be more fully in charge in her second sport: 'I've become something of a control freak. In the past, once or twice I allowed people to help me who didn't actually have my best interests at heart. There are ways in which you're just a number in someone else's big business model, and you can't just hand over your career, you need to know why decisions are being made. There are some younger athletes around the squad at the moment who are probably less involved in their own careers than they think they are.'

There's something else, of course. Everything I've said so far about being an athlete is limited in scope. I've talked about the bits where you're obviously on the payroll. The really difficult thing to deal with for many is this: everything you do will make you faster or make you slower. This isn't just everything you do from a training point of view, or even an eating point of view, but everything from an everything point of view. Because an athlete makes their living with their body, everything they do to or with it, everywhere they take it, and everything they put in it has some consequence. It might be an immeasurably small consequence, but there is nothing that is neither 'good' nor 'bad'. Marginal gain or marginal guilt – your choice.

All the time you ask yourself, 'Will it make me tired. Is there any risk I'll pick up an injury? Will I get an infection?' These are reasons to avoid standing up, walking, and staying awake. Or leaving the house for any purpose other than training.

I once went five years without going to the cinema. It wasn't that big a sacrifice – my body fat was sufficiently low that the lack of padding on my arse meant I couldn't sit still for long enough to watch a film all the way through anyway. I missed weddings – not just the ones I didn't want to go to (almost all of them) but the handful I really wanted to be at. Only rarely was there a clash with an actual race – normally it was just fear of getting a cold or giving myself tendonitis by dancing (very easy to do). When two of my best friends got married, the date of the wedding was planned to suit me. Not them.

In case you think it's just me that behaves like this, Chris Boardman missed the birth of his second child to go and recce the course for a national TT championships. Not actually ride the race or anything. Just go and look at the roads. It was, I suppose, a question of priorities.

I didn't mind this sort of thing all that much. If you have the feeling that I'm not the sort of man who regrets too deeply being unable to spend his weekend evenings compacted into a pub full of shoulders and elbows so that I can shout 'no, really, just a still mineral water please' into a variety of badly cleaned ears, then you'd be right. There are riders for whom it's something they badly miss, something that makes them unhappy and resentful.

This is when it gets complicated. Here's the equation: if I go out, there is a 5% risk I'll catch a cold, and a 3% risk I'll get tendonitis. There is a 15% reduction in the effectiveness of my recovery from the previous day's session, and a 20% reduction in the commitment I'll be able to summon up for the following day. There is a 30% risk I'll fall off the wagon and get bladdered, whereupon I might as well not have done most of the previous week at all. However, I'm also sick to the back teeth of living like a monk. If I don't have a night out, have a bit of a release, see some people who don't spend their whole lives worrying about their lactate thresholds and, what's worse, talking about it, there is a 50% risk I'll get so pissed off that all motivation will cease, and the quality of everything I do will enter a decline. There is a 3% risk that things will get so bad I'll either give up competitive cycling, or get fired by the team at the end of the season. Jesus, I need a drink.

I've heard one or two riders refer to the odd night out as 'morale training'. It's a good expression for it. It's got the word 'training' in it, so it's got to be a good idea.

That equation is not the end of it. The aim of a professional athlete is to reduce life to training, eating, and recovering – sitting about. The sitting about is deadly. At a training camp you can feel your life dribbling through your fingers. You can walk round the hotel and find riders in corners making endless Skype calls, playing video games, watching films, or just staring blankly into space waiting for the next excuse to get on a bike. I wrote my first book because of the sitting about. I think it was either that or learn the guitar, and I thought the book would annoy people less.

Stresses stack up, wherever they come from. The hormones involved create physical effects – so the boiler breaking down disrupts your recovery. The aim of a training camp is to eliminate all the bits of home life that might marginally get in the way. No cooking, no shopping, no bills to pay, no one round for dinner. No promises to keep. In an ideal world you'd eliminate everything from home as well. You'd regress to a second infancy, one with even less stress than the first one. Ride, eat, drowse your way through half a movie, and sleep.

It's hard to ride seriously and hold down a job, even where the job is essentially sedentary. You'd think being a writer would be ideal – I mean, it's basically indistinguishable from sitting about. It's better than most, but it's hard to be a good writer and a good athlete at the same time. The energy seems to come from the same place. I know several retired riders who've agreed that a normal day's work is exhausting. A lot of them abandon bike riding immediately the pay-cheques stop because they struggle to find the time and enthusiasm as soon as cycling has to fit round life rather than life fit round cycling. Most, eventually, come back to it. Usually not long after they realise they can no longer see their feet.

I'm going to go out on a limb here, and make a suggestion that I have only anecdotal evidence to support. I think that for a lot of professional bike riders, there is a progression to their relationship with their sport. It starts when they are young, and they ride a bike, and they love it. They like riding fast. They like swishing round corners. They like the feeling. They enter their first race, and most of them either win, or very nearly win, because almost nobody who's on the way to becoming an elite rider is a turkey first time out.

Competition becomes more important. A new world beckons, one of racing and training and looking for the small gains and worrying about the details. Websites and magazines are trawled with care. A coach appears, either sought out by a rider or their parents, or just as likely, the coach comes looking for the rider. The degree of serious-ness takes another step up.

This is the point where it becomes about being an athlete, rather than about being a bike rider. They enjoy the process. The relationship with the coach, being part of a team. Watching themselves improve, developing a career. Competing. Winning. And most of all they enjoy having found something they are good at.

To go back to Dowsett for a moment. I interviewed him in a well-known cyclists' cafe in Essex on a Wednesday morning. He'd ridden the hour over from home. The place was filled with Essex bike riders, many of them of a certain age, stopping to refuel on a ride. 'Something I don't often say, in case people take it the wrong way,' said Dowsett, 'but look around. This place is full of people who just love riding, love getting out on their bikes for a few miles. Most pros aren't like that. There are a few, but not very many, and I'm not one of them. I don't enjoy the training very much. But I love racing. I love winning. Most of all, I've found something I'm very good at, and I very much enjoy being very good at it.'

It's dangerously easy to give the impression that the rarefied world of elite sport is a terrible place. 'It's hard.' 'It demands everything you have.' 'You give it your whole life – everything you do is part of your sport, part of your career.' 'You won't see the inside of a nightclub till you're so old that the music will have become that same indescribable racket your dad used to complain about every time you switched on Radio 1.' The things that are most easily articulated are those that make it all sound like a punishment, and my own accounts are more guilty of that than most.

The thing that no one talks about enough is the sheer pleasure of it. When I was at the height of my abilities, there were moments when the only way I could describe what it was like was to say I felt the way a thoroughbred horse looks at full gallop. There is a balance and a rhythm that is both irresistible and effortless. Like a galloping horse, every bit of you is part of the motion, even the bits that are quite still. The involvement, physically and mentally, is total, because you've trained all of you for this one task, and you've had the purity of purpose in your life to do it without compromises. Everything you've ever done comes to a single point. For a few moments you feel quite perfect.

Winning is nice. When you're a young athlete it's a thrill, when you're an old athlete it's a relief, and it's no less wonderful for that. It can pay the bills. It can certainly justify your time and your career, because winning is the only negotiable currency in the world of sport. Winning reassures everyone that you are not wasting your life, it makes it clear that you are good at what you do. But winning isn't as much of a joy as that feeling of balance and rhythm. By the end of a career, winning will quite probably be something you can take or leave, because you'll have learned that winning isn't something you can control. It's the perfection you'll be desperate to feel one last time.

I'm aware there's an arrogance about what I'm saying, because I'm suggesting that sport at the elite level is different in its kind, not just in its speed. Perhaps it's not quite that black and white. But there is something about the dedication of whole years of existence to a single physical goal that I think does make it special. It's what you're for.

There are things that are less visceral. There is satisfaction in getting towards the top of any field. There is pleasure in both the collaboration of a team, and the solitary focus of an individual rider. There are days when, despite everything going wrong, you still manage to fight back for something that you can be proud of, even if it goes unnoticed by anyone else.

You can go for an easy recovery ride, one of the times you might take a moment to look at the hedges and the fields, and find yourself smiling at the idea that your recovery ride has become faster than you were once able to race. There is even something rather nice about the feeling of deep-down tiredness that swamps you after some hard races or training sessions. You can paste yourself to the sofa with the feeling, right there in your legs, of a job done well.

Parts of an athlete's life are hard, yes. But having the chance to dedicate yourself to something that's both so extraordinary and so unnecessary means it's also rather wonderful.

CHAPTER 2

Blood, oxygen and muscle: the physiology of an athlete

THERE IS A STORY THAT AT A BRITISH TIME TRIAL EVENT IN the 1970s, one of the discipline's grand champions was asked by a well-beaten rival just what the secret was. Why was he so good? Why could he do what no one else could? Was it a training session no one else had stumbled upon? Was it a special way of pedalling? Was it psychological? There had to be ... something. Something that made him different.

The grand champion said he would show him. He led him over to his bike and pointed at one of the pedals. His rival bent down to give it a close examination. 'You see that? Well, when that little bastard gets to the top, I kick it to the bottom as hard as I'm able. When it gets to the top again, I do the same thing. And I keep doing it.'

This is pretty much the secret.

Cycling is a sport of details, of tactics, technology, training and psychology. But before it is any of those things, it is a sport that depends on how hard you can turn the pedals. This is the absolute basic. However obvious it might appear, almost everyone involved in cycling manages to forget it at some point.

Ours is a sport that is intensely physiological. There is not much technique, not really. The bike, the wheels, the helmet, they all make some difference. Maybe at the top level they make a significant difference. But zoom out to the big picture, and the details become just details and what matters is all about force through the pedals. That's what distinguishes the stars from the also-rans, and the also-rans from those who didn't even make it to the race. Cycling may well be the most physically unforgiving sport there is.

The fundamental differences between individuals can be pretty large. Sir Bradley Wiggins won the British ten-mile time-trial championships in 2011 – one of his relatively few appearances at a UK domestic race. I'm picking on this race because the field was not of big-name pros, but consisted of riders from Wiggins down to good domestic club riders – people with some talent who take the sport reasonably seriously but who aren't professionals, and certainly aren't global stars.

Wiggins won the event in 19'14". I was second in 19'55", which was less of an embarrassment than I was expecting, but that's not where I'm going with this. The rider in 93rd place did 24'03". For him to have ridden as fast as Wiggins would have required him to find something around twice the power he actually produced. Clearly there are some other issues around that – aerodynamics being the main one – but it's still a daunting margin. Ride as hard as you possibly can. You're halfway there.

If 93rd seems a bit too distant to be relevant, well, here's another way of looking at it. Wiggins' average power for the ride was about 470w. He could still have made the top 20 on 334w. For Wiggins, 334w is easy training pace. Given enough fuel, he could do it almost indefinitely. Five to six hours would certainly not be any kind of a problem, and he could do it while holding a conversation that was in no way compromised by having to breathe anywhere that there wasn't a comma. But it's still good enough to beat some relatively serious bike riders.

On the other hand, Wiggins, flat out in a sprint, would probably not manage any more than 1,200w (this is an educated guess – these aren't the kind of numbers that get handed out too readily). A track sprinter of the Sir Chris Hoy variety can hit something over 2,300w – not only that, but he can do it from a standing start, which Wiggins certainly couldn't. Hoy, in turn, would quite probably struggle to finish twentieth in the ten-mile championships. Neither could beat Mark Cavendish in a big bunch sprint on the road. And none of these three, not even Wiggins, would live with a full-blooded attack by a pure climber in the high mountains.

And all three are, in their own way, much, much finer examples of kicking the bastard pedals around than 99.99% of the rest of us.

Understanding how an athlete can do what they can do starts with their basic physiology. I want to ignore, for the moment, the issues of how they come to have that physiology in the first place, or how they would set about trying to change aspects of it that aren't as good as they might be. I'll get to that later. For now, I just want to look at exactly what an athlete is.

My first attempts to understand all of this came when I started working with the exercise physiologist Jamie Pringle. Ten years ago, he called me out of the blue one afternoon to see if there was any physiological support he could offer during an attempt I made on the world hour record. It says a lot about how much the sport has changed in the decade since that up till then I hadn't even thought to look for any scientific backup – indeed I didn't even have a coach at that point, having parted company with the GB squad coach who'd been looking after me up till then.

When Jamie tested me in the lab – an exhilarating world of stationary bikes, breathing masks, rubber gloves and blood samples – I was genuinely astonished at the results. Despite displaying a fairly clear talent for riding a bike, it hadn't occurred to me – or indeed to anyone else – that I was anything special. The first announcement of my abilities came from a machine, and frankly, being told you're brilliant is an experience that is only enhanced by that kind of objectivity.

The machine in question, merely the first of many adoring pieces of lab equipment to which Jamie introduced me, was one that measured lung capacity. You blew into a hose, and a pen drew a line on a bit of graph paper (it was an endearingly analogue machine). I blew the pen off the top of the graph in the most literal sense. I could tell that was unusual, because there were no other lines on the machine's plastic case. I managed to expel just under eight litres, which for someone of my height (180cm) is, in all modesty, phenomenal. I had a peak ventilation rate – just how much you can breathe in and out in a minute – of around 230 litres. As Jamie put it, I was in horse territory. If riding a bike didn't work out, I would clearly have a vocation as an assistant to a balloon-animal maker.*

The big-ticket number in these things is VO_2 max – a concept that has entered common parlance among those bike riders who tend even slightly towards the geeky. It's simply the maximum amount of oxygen you can use in a minute. You find it by means of a torture that consists of riding a stationary bike at a pace that increases relentlessly until eventually your body screams that it can pedal no

---

* A couple of years later, while researching a book on sailing, I blew up a rubber dinghy by mouth in ten minutes. I almost passed out.

more and you collapse over the handlebars. While you're riding, a physiologist measures how much oxygen you're using via a mask and an expensive machine. The biggest number that flits across the screen is your VO_2 max. You can keep going, and ride faster than VO_2 max pace – albeit not for all that long – but you won't be able to use any more oxygen to do so. It's your maximum aerobic capacity, or the size of your aerobic motor, in millilitres of oxygen per minute per kilo of body weight. Think of it like the cubic capacity of a car engine.

An average untrained man of my age would have a VO_2 max of around 40ml/m/kg. Training effects vary by individual, but an average for a decent club athlete would be something like 60. I hit 85. A year later I hit 90, which was higher than any other cyclist any of us had ever heard of. There have been a handful who've topped that since, but you could probably count them on your fingers.

(It's worth saying that reliable numbers are sometimes difficult to find because physiological studies of professional sportsmen have been badly corrupted over the years by the doping problem. Some numbers may be trustworthy, some certainly aren't. The numbers provided for Lance Armstrong were widely agreed to be implausible because they were too modest. He simply wouldn't have been able to go as fast as he did if the study numbers were all he'd been able to do. If you took the lab results at face value, I should have been faster than him. Somewhere between the lab and the road he'd apparently found a second heart and some extra blood. Which was at least half true.)

I didn't really know what to make of all this. In a basic way it answered the question of why I was so fast on a bike: I had a very big engine. But, if you're at all inquisitive, that was where a lot more questions began. What was the key to it? Was it just lung capacity? Or was it more complicated?

But there was a more pressing question. If I was that good in the lab, why was I not a much better bike rider in the real world than I actually was? And was knowing more detail about how I functioned going to lead me to something I could do that would reduce that discrepancy?

There are no simple answers to any of this. Human physiology is so complicated that I find myself regularly regarding it as a proof against the theory of intelligent design, on the basis that absolutely no one would have set about designing something that was so convoluted, contradictory, and just plain messy. Like a taxation system, it swirls with bits apparently slapped on at random to fix a loophole that no one saw coming, with widely differing solutions to apparently similar problems deployed according to no criteria that are obvious. It is chaos in there. How we've made sense of what we've learned so far baffles me, and there is plenty of weirdness left to go.

The scale of the differences between individuals are perhaps most astonishing of all. For anyone who's interested in physiology in elite sport and wants to push performance forward, it's these variances that are important. The average abilities of a large population are interesting, but other than giving you a basic benchmark, or a warm glow of unearned superiority, they're of little help.

Even the averages of an elite group of athletes in the same sport don't tell you all that much. What you really want to know is not that an athlete is extraordinary, but exactly how they're extraordinary, because there are quite a few different ways to excel at the same thing. VO_2 max is great as a single-figure guide, especially for physiologists, because it's quite stable from day to day – it doesn't depend on how hard an athlete tries. But in the real world, its usefulness is diminished by a host of other variables. If you want to perform better, you need to know precisely what's holding you back, and that's not necessarily the same thing that's holding someone else back.

Let's slip away from bike riding for a moment, and into marathon running, which as a sport is approaching the headline-breakthrough of the sub-two-hour run. (I'm using it because it's the kind of objective record that cycling generally lacks.) To do it would take a runner with a VO_2 max of about 92ml/m/kg, with the ability to run at about 85% of that effort level for the race. They'd also need to be highly efficient in the way they combine that oxygen with fuel and turn it into forward motion, around 180ml/kg for every kilometre covered. To extend the earlier car-engine metaphor, this means that the athlete would have to have a large capacity, the ability to run for two hours at almost maximum revs, and to produce power efficiently.

These numbers are not impossible, or even extremely rare. In the UK alone there are several runners with one of these characteristics, and a few with two. No one in the world has yet managed to combine all three.

As a road time-trial rider, my concerns were very similar to those of a marathon runner. It was all about endurance physiology and aerobic conditioning. The issue of sprint physiology, anaerobic energy, was still an element of what I was doing, but a sufficiently marginal one that it was never where I went looking for gains. My career was unusually pure: most competitive bike riding involves a much more flexible combination of aerobic and anaerobic. On the road, attacks and sprints have an anaerobic component, as do short prologues and team time trials. All track events have at least some element of sprinting to them. But I'm going to start with what I'm good at, and that's moving and using oxygen.

I'm going to attempt to explain what goes on during exercise via a practical demonstration. There are a number

of standard lab-test protocols to which physiologists enjoy
subjecting athletes. The second-least pleasant of these is
called a ramp test – we'll get to the least pleasant one a little
later. The details are from a test I did a few seasons ago,
selected more or less at random from a year when both
Jamie and I were trying to keep a close track of the changes
to my physiology over the course of a racing season, and
consequently did a lot of lab work. I also admit that, from
an ego-massage point of view, it's one of my better tests.

The protocol was a simple one. I started pedalling on a
stationary bike at a power output of 200w. Every 15
seconds, the power required edged up by five watts. This
happened automatically. This ramp continued until I was
no longer able to keep going – the point of failure or
exhaustion. Throughout, my pulse was recorded and my
expired breath went to a gas-analysis machine that kept
track of what I was breathing out, and hence what was
happening to the air in my lungs. Every minute a blood
sample was taken from my thumb, and analysed for lactate
concentration. You may know lactate better as 'lactic acid'
– it's produced in the muscles, especially during intense
exercise, and its concentration in the blood is used to define
some important landmarks. It's measured in millimoles per
millilitre. That's the closest to biochemistry we're going to
get. There's no need at all to know what it means, but I
have to call it something.

The ramp-test starting point of 200w is dead easy – for
me it was below even recovery pace. The only thing
stopping me from trying to continue a conversation was
the breathing mask. My pulse at that point was just under
120bpm – beats per minute – equivalent to not much more
than walking. I was using 2.4 litres of oxygen a minute. The
lactate level was 1.1mmol/ml, actually slightly lower than
my resting lactate level.

Five minutes later, at 300w, all that had moved on to a pulse of 142bpm, oxygen uptake to 3.5 litres, and lactate remained at a constant 1.1mmol/ml. 300w is still pretty easy – at that point in the season it was less than my long ride (four- to five-hour) average.

Here, roughly, is what's happening. Each breath takes air to the lungs. You don't replace the whole contents of your lungs with each breath, so the air there has less oxygen than fresh air – in the depths of the lung it's about 14.5% oxygen compared to 20.1% for the air outside, with carbon dioxide accounting for the difference.

Oxygen diffuses into the blood simply because (even at 14.5%) it is more concentrated in the air of the lung than it is in the blood – it's pushed by a pressure gradient. Carbon dioxide diffuses in the opposite direction, again because of the difference in concentration. The exchange of gases is very, very fast – it takes about a quarter of a second to complete. At rest, that's about a third of the time it takes the blood to pass through the lungs. Even if you're racing at full stretch, it doesn't change very much because the blood vessels transiting the lung increase in volume to allow a higher throughput of blood without much increase in its actual speed. Blood will take as much oxygen as it can hold from the normal concentration of oxygen in the lungs – you wouldn't get any more by breathing pure oxygen.

Contrary to what you might expect, a very great deal of endurance ability is not in the lungs, or the muscles, but in the blood. How much oxygen the blood can move round the body is critical. Just how critical you can judge from the phenomenal amount of time, money, inconvenience, risk, drug-test dodging and generalised dishonesty that has gone into illicitly improving it over the last couple of decades. There are two main issues: the quantity of oxygen a given amount of blood can carry, and how much blood you have in total.

The first question depends on the amount of haemoglobin you've got, since that's what carries the oxygen, and that depends on the number of red blood cells you have. If you use a centrifuge to separate out the different elements of blood, you find that the average for a given quantity of ordinary, non-athletic blood is about 46% red cells for men and 40% for women. This percentage is called the haematocrit.

The variation is quite large – for men 42 to 52% would be unremarkable. But in endurance athletes, it's a few percentage points less, because endurance training alters the composition of the blood. Most non-sprint riders have the rather dramatically titled, but basically harmless, condition of athletic anaemia: their blood is diluted by a greater than normal amount of plasma, the liquid in which all the cells bob about. The increase in plasma occurs within a few days of starting regular training, and can be quite large.

The changes don't end there. Over the next three to four weeks of training the total number of red cells will rise as well, though it doesn't usually match the increase in plasma. The eventual result is a greater amount of slightly less concentrated blood, but with a net increase in the total number of red cells. Since more blood is good, and more red cells are even better, the overall effect is that more oxygen can be carried. Blood plasma will also fall very fast when you stop training. It's the reason for most of the drop off you see, especially the increase in pulse at any given level of effort after a couple of weeks' break from training. And the rapid increase back to 'athlete-normal' plasma volume is why the first session back after a short break will be horrendous, the second will be bad, and the third will be almost the same as before the break.

There were riders in the 1980s and 1990s who took the process a very major step beyond what they'd get by mere training, and illegally boosted their haematocrit from what you'd expect at around 42–44% to over 60%, and in one particularly outstanding example 73%, either by using EPO to stimulate red-cell production or by simply infusing red cells. The relationship between red-cell count and carrying oxygen is a pretty direct one. One study found that an increase in haematocrit from 43% to 54% produced a huge 13% increase in VO_2 max. Blood doping is not something that makes some sort of footling, marginal difference to performance. It's taking your body back to the shop and exchanging it for a much, much better one. It's far beyond anything you could achieve with better training.

EPO is actually a naturally occurring hormone, which stimulates the production of red blood cells. Until the last decade it was impossible to distinguish the synthetic drug version from the natural version, and it's still not easy. The authorities' only recourse was a sort of clampdown that comprised taking blood samples from riders, testing them and making sure they didn't surpass a specified maximum haematocrit of 50%.

This was described as a 'health measure', because very high red-cell content made the blood thick and strawberry-jam-esque, and very hard for the heart to pump. Every so often an athlete would die from a mysterious heart failure, generally at night when the blood flow was slow. There were stories in the 1990s of athletes getting up in the middle of the night to jog up and down hotel corridors to get the blood moving a bit.

A haematocrit value of over 50% was not a dope-test fail. The rider would be withdrawn from competition until his blood values had 'returned to normal' – make of that what you will. 50% was still quite a lot more than usual for an endurance rider, so a more cynical view would be that it was not so much a deterrent to cheating, as a limit to how much you could cheat. It also gave an advantage to a doper with a naturally low haematocrit, because they had more headroom for boosting their blood quality before they ran into the limit.

Numerous riders have explained how they worked to keep their cell-count at the limit. Part of the fall-out from the Lance Armstrong case was testimony that teams would give riders 'emergency' infusions of plasma to dilute the blood if they suspected a test was imminent, and even stall for time when the testers arrived at a team hotel to allow the procedure to take place.

The second element of the blood equation is not quality, but sheer quantity. Setting aside anything illicit, you might be lucky, and just naturally have buckets of the stuff. Many endurance athletes do. The average 75kg man has a blood volume of around 6 litres. Exercise will increase this to maybe 6.5 litres. Me? I've got 9.5 litres. Some riders the same size might get to 11 litres. It's one of the key markers. It doesn't take much imagination to see that a huge amount of blood pumping through the lungs will allow the collection of a very great deal of oxygen, and oxygen is what the game is about.

You can achieve something similar by simply popping some more in from a blood bag, of the sort you see on medical dramas, and which many teams covertly smuggled all over the world. This is, of course, against the rules. It was an undetectable practice until relatively recently. The initial reaction of one of the first riders to be snared by the new test was rumoured to have been, 'Really? But I didn't think there was a test for that!' He went on to deny everything for several years, before the inevitable reveal-all book deal.

It's the blood that carries the oxygen, but the blood can only deliver it to the muscles because it's pumped round the body by the heart. That brings us to a rather good experiment. In 1992 a team of scientists from San Diego acquired a group of racing pigs. Pig racing happens in several US states, generally in areas where the audience hasn't been tempted away by subsidised opera. It's a fairly simple concept: you take pigs, you make them race. It's usually state-fair material rather than ESPN.

The team made the pigs run to exhaustion on a treadmill – essentially the same ramp test as I do. (There is almost nothing that hasn't been made to run on a treadmill at some point, from horses to lobsters. With horses you need a special harness so you can hoist them off the treadmill before they gallop themselves to death. This proves that lobsters are smarter than horses.) They found those pigs which had had the substantial pericardium membrane that surrounds the heart loosened showed very impressive improvements, namely that their oxygen uptake improved by a whopping average of 31%.

The pericardium is not there for decorative purposes, it's there to stabilise and protect the heart. The prognosis for the experiment group of pigs was not, therefore, as bright as you would hope. The interesting thing is that it also restricts the size of the heart and so its ability to pump. What the experiment showed was that if you increased the size of the pump, you immediately increased the effectiveness of the aerobic system. The pumping capacity of the heart is the single most important part of the endurance athlete package. Unsurprisingly I've heard the suggestion that the next generation of doping products are likely to focus round the heart and the elasticity of the pericardium, rather than the current target, the quality of the blood.

Even without such dubious interventions, serious athletes have good hearts. At rest, an average-sized man, whether trained or not, needs to pump about five litres of blood a minute to keep everything running. Untrained, the pulse rate that sustains this is around 70bpm. Trained, it's more like 50, perhaps lower. (Sub 40bpm is not all that unusual, and sub 30 is not entirely unknown. Mine, at its lowest, was about 35bpm.) Simple maths shows that the volume of blood that squirts out with each pulse is about 50% higher in an 'average' elite athlete, and for some, like me, it's even more.

This greater volume-per-pulse – the cardiac stroke volume – is related to the increase in blood plasma that comes with greater fitness. The extra plasma prompts an increase in the size of the heart's left ventricle, as well as increasing the flexibility of both the heart and the arteries.

This extra volume becomes a lot more important when not at rest, because the maximum pulse of trained and untrained will not be all that different. At that point, say 200bpm, the next bit of simple maths shows that the athletes can move 50% more blood per minute. In practice it actually comes in a bit higher, like 60%. To put an actual number on it, that's likely to mean an athlete pumping 35 litres of blood a minute, which is the same as a bath tap turned full on. That's compared to an average club rider who would be around 20 litres, or the 'sedentary' group, whose role it is to prop up the bottom of all these kinds of statistics, with about 15. How much your heart can pump is very closely related to your VO_2 max. It is also the single most dramatic change brought about by endurance training.

Everything up to here has been relatively straightforward. How the oxygen gets into the blood is, conceptually at least, fairly simple. How the blood then gets to the muscle is just plumbing. Heavy breathing, pulse elevated, job done. How the oxygen gets out of the blood, combines with fuel, and turns the bastard pedals is more involved.

The transition starts with blood vessels. Take 'em all out and put them end to end, and you'll find that there are about 100,000 miles worth of them in your common or garden elite bike rider. Most of this extravagant pipework is the capillaries, the very tiny blood vessels that run through the muscle to each individual muscle fibre. I mean tiny – there are between 200 and 500 of them to each square millimetre of muscle cross-section. Like almost everything else in the system, these are different in athletes – there are about 40% more of them than the non-athlete average. And the number of them that are active at any one time changes: under hard riding, the number increases about 30-fold, which means that despite the higher speed at which the blood leaves the heart, it passes through the muscle at a fairly constant rate, just over a wider area.

Skeletal muscle, the sort we use for movement, is made up of bundles of parallel muscle fibres, a bit like a handful of drinking straws. Each fibre – straw – contains countless tiny parallel rods called myofibrils, each composed of shorter rods called sarcomeres, which contain a further, and thankfully final, set of even smaller parallel rods called myofilaments. These are the things that do the actual contracting, like microscopic trombone-slides.

They do this in response to a molecule called adenosine triphosphate, known as ATP. I remember my biology teacher at school talking about this stuff for lessons on end, while I ignored her completely on the basis that the biology of muscular contraction was clearly not something in which I would ever have the slightest interest. I only remembered the name because I continually got the initials confused with those of the Advanced Passenger Train, an abject transport failure from a few years previously, but which was still a lot more interesting than ATP.

I would probably ignore it even now, but it's hard to avoid, since without it, the muscle won't function. There is very, very little of it about at any given moment – the total in the body is just a few grams. But it's constantly created in the muscle. It's this ATP manufacture that all that oxygen moving was working towards.

Before I embarked on the crash-course in the entire human cardiovascular system that we've just gone through, I was last seen undertaking that ramp test. The pace was a nice steady one, with a pulse of 140bpm and a power output of 300w. At this stage almost all of the ATP was being made from oxygen combining with energy from fat and carbohydrate. The reaction of oxygen with hydrogen from the fuel formed water as a waste product, which is released into the bloodstream to become sweat, urine, or the condensation in exhaled breath. This is a steady state of equilibrium, and a nice moderate pace for bike riding. The only reason I couldn't have kept doing it indefinitely is that I'd run out of fuel. Even so, that would probably only happen quite a long time after I got bored.

A minute further on, at 143bpm and 325w, I got to the first of the physiological landmarks: lactate threshold. Up to this point there was a low, consistent background of lactate in my blood, around 1.1mmol/ml. At 325w, this started to increase with each incremental step up in riding intensity. (A club racer would probably hit this change at about 200w.)

Lactate comes about because, as well as the ATP that's produced aerobically from oxygen combining with fat and carbohydrate, some ATP is made anaerobically, without oxygen. For that ATP, the hydrogen can't combine with oxygen to make water. Instead it produces lactate.

Lactate is produced in the muscles from anaerobic production of ATP all the time, even when you're at rest. It's cleared from the bloodstream on an equally constant basis. But production of lactate increases as effort levels go up, and lactate threshold is the point at which this increase starts to become evident. The threshold is not a particularly major change of gear. Even at these higher concentrations, the lactate is still cleared as fast as it's produced, so the intensities at and just above lactate threshold remain, physiologically, steady state. That is, for any level of effort, the lactate concentration will stay the same, and it will only increase if you ride harder. For me, in this test, as the intensity edged up past the threshold, lactate went up to 2.5mmol/ml or so.

As a riding intensity, lactate threshold isn't all that hard. You wouldn't want to deliver a lecture on aerobic metabolism at the same time, but on a bike, or in the lab, it's a perfectly doable pace. For me, lactate threshold has got mainly to do with setting training intensities, and particularly monitoring what effects the training is having. The first thing that moves as I start to get fitter is lactate threshold.

For this, it helps very much that for a lot of riders it's associated with a clear break in the breathing rhythm. If I ride at a steadily increasing intensity, I find there's a step change in the rhythm as the effort increases. It's even more obvious if I go running, where breathing and stride pattern are in sync. I can tell where my lactate threshold is just from the way I'm breathing, which in terms of tracking condition is a huge bonus.

From this point on in the ramp test, lactate levels increase with every step up in intensity. Each minute, each 20w, becomes quite noticeable. It's still controlled, though. Breathing is steady, moderately quick, but relaxed. My pace for a 100-mile time trial is in this area somewhere, and that's a three-and-a-half hour effort.

Still, it's not long until you get to the most significant landmark of all. You'd think, given the importance of this one, that the physiologists would have come up with a snappy name for it. But they've called it the Onset of Blood Lactate Accumulation. Or OBLA, for short.*

Up to this point, the elevated lactate level will still stabilise at a given level of effort. Beyond this, even if the effort level stays the same, the amount of lactate begins to increase exponentially. OBLA for a club rider would probably be around 275w. In my case, in this test, OBLA happened at 400w, pretty much exactly, and a pulse of 164bpm. Lactate concentration was 4mmol/ml. (A pulse of 164bpm at this point was rather low for me. In other tests it was more normally around 170bpm.)

OBLA is key to endurance sport, because it's the maximum pace you can maintain for sustained periods, up to about an hour. And, indeed, later in that same lab session I did a 60-minute trial at 400w, which was stupendously boring, but otherwise manageable. During it my heart rate drifted up to the low 170s, which happens in sustained efforts, partly due to fluid loss in sweat depleting your blood volume slightly. My lactate level during the long trial stayed nicely balanced on the upper threshold of steady state, around 3.8mmol/ml. Only a few watts more would have seen it start to climb inexorably.

There is a second breathing breakpoint in a ramp test, which coincides, give or take a bit, with OBLA. It's the point where breathing becomes fast. For a runner, it's

---

* I blame the decline of the classical education. Once, they'd have said this in Latin, and it would have sounded a lot more professional for it. The terminology is actually the subject of a lot of debate. Some coaches and physiologists insist that OBLA should really be called Maximum Lactate Steady State (MLSS), some the Second Lactate Turnpoint. A lot of them use 'OBLA' to mean a specific lactate concentration of 4mmol/ml, which is not how I'm using it here. There are several other, even more cumbersome and/or misleading descriptions. Once upon a time it was called the 'Anaerobic Threshold', long abandoned on the basis that it simply didn't describe what was happening. There isn't really a good, universal term for it. I'm sticking to OBLA because it's the name I'm familiar with.

breathing every stride, and for a cyclist, it's the same fast, consistent rhythm. As with lactate threshold, I can usually judge OBLA fairly accurately by my breathing rate. Given the practical significance of OBLA as a sustainable race pace this is a very useful talent.

Past OBLA is where a ramp test starts to get hard. The effort is not sustainable, and life just gets progressively more and more unpleasant. Like a race, it's not painful, not as such, you just have to concentrate on keeping the pace high and staying as relaxed as you can, and blocking out the urge to stop. Anywhere north of OBLA, whether I'm racing, training or lab testing, I focus on breathing – breathing rhythm is always at the heart of how I gauge an effort.

I need to keep my pedalling cadence high at these power levels. Ideally I want to stay up round 120rpm, maybe 130. As the test enters its endgame, my breathing rate hits its maximum, and I realise I'm in sprinters' territory, not mine. Even when I'm getting towards the end, and wind up for a final finishing effort, it doesn't feel the way I know a sprint should. There's no extra gear, no explosive finish, just a last lurch against the inevitable. Out with a quite literal whimper. Lactate this time topped out at about 9mmol/ml. In other tests I've seen levels up round 13 or 14 – perhaps for this test I was a little tired.

Still, the point of failure, of giving up, always takes me a little by surprise when it arrives. My legs stop without me. I'm always certain I could, and should, have done more, if only I'd been prepared to try harder. I'm wrong, though. The absolute values at failure change, but if you look at it relative only to my own physiology, it's actually exactly the same every time. I always try to the same level of 'hard'. When I get to within a couple of minutes of the end, and my breathing rate starts to hit its limit, Jamie (who almost invariably runs the test) can look at the data on his screen and predict how much I've got left almost to the second. The variation in my ramp test results is always down to underlying physical ability, rather than motivation.

The last marker passed on the way to my vision going black and white is the one we've already mentioned, VO_2 max, the maximum oxygen uptake. It occurs quite near the end, because oxygen uptake still keeps increasing after the anaerobic mechanisms start to play a more significant role at OBLA. In this particular test, VO_2 max was 6.2 litres/m, or 85.5ml/m/kg, and occurred at 528w. The failure point was about 45 seconds or 15w beyond that. As a physiological profile for an elite endurance athlete, it was a pretty good test. The numbers at the top end were impressive, especially the VO_2 max figure.

The more important numbers were further back, though. They're the ones that show why I was unlikely to translate that monster engine into an Olympic medal. One issue was that I wasn't very efficient – while my VO_2 max was world class, the actual horsepower I was making with all that oxygen was unspectacular, at least in comparison to the elite riders I wanted to beat.

The second and bigger issue was that the proportion of my maximum that I could sustain was average by any measure. Top riders can manage to hold 85%, occasionally even 90% of their VO_2 max power. I was doing only 74%, which is about what you'd expect from an average club rider. It was unspectacular in comparison to the customers at a cyclists' cafe on a Sunday morning. If I'd been able to hang on to a sustained percentage that was in line with the rest of my profile, OBLA – and my sustainable riding pace – would have been around 450w. That's about 2kph faster than what I could do. If I could have done that … well, I'd have been amazing. But I couldn't. And even I'm smart enough to be grateful for the rest of the test profile.

This test was a typical one – I have dozens of test result files that tell the same story of patchy glory. Great heart, good blood, and an OBLA that still happens too early. The hunch was that this was probably down to what was going on at the further reaches of the cardiovascular system – especially the density of capillaries and the delivery of oxygen deep within the muscles.

Over the subsequent couple of seasons, I did manage to get the sustainable percentage of max up, at least a bit. But simultaneously my efficiency went down, leaving only a small net improvement. Over a still longer span, up to much more recent times, the proportion did go up to 80% or so – but only because VO_2 max went down. It was an unsquareable circle. But we did at least focus on the things that were most likely to make a difference. I went faster for knowing what was slowing me down.

It's only reasonable to admit that part of the reason the numbers were as impressive as they were over all was because I'm a terrific lab rat. I love it in there. I get as big a thrill from posting big numbers in the lab as I do from winning races. Cracking 90ml/m/kg for a VO_2 max score ranks as one of my best moments in bike riding. I am well aware of the contempt in which most sane bike racers will hold me for this, and they are quite right to do so. It's the missing-the-point equivalent of a hi-fi buff who stands you on a cross on his carpet to enjoy a perfect, undistorted, beautifully stereo-imaged rendition of Steps' Greatest Hits.

My lab-test advantages extend beyond mere enthusiasm. I'm a very pure endurance athlete, and lab tests are historically very good at dealing with people like me. It's a real chance to shine. In contrast, on the basis of his lab tests at British Cycling in the early 2000s, Mark Cavendish was all but told he'd got no hope as a professional bike racer. One of the coaches of whom Cavendish was later most critical was the same one who retained quite a close interest in what I was doing long after it was clear that, on the track at least (the main concern at BC at the time) I was not an Olympic medal prospect.

That's not the only respect in which I'm the anti-Cavendish. It's not so much that I'm a bad sprinter as that I'm no sprinter at all. For years there was an unkind rumour that at my first national squad lab assessment, after I'd done the sprint test the coach said, 'Yes, just like that, but actually sprint this time.' This isn't true. He knew I was sprinting. I knew he knew because I could hear him sniggering.

A more embarrassing illustration of my sprinting absence-of-prowess was at a bike show, where one of the stands had a knock-out sprint competition set up on two stationary bikes. I was browbeaten into doing it by a friend who was running the stand. I changed into my cycling kit and shoes, and insisted they install my preferred brand of pedal on my bike. (This wasn't arrogance; it was because I was trying to mitigate the imminent humiliation.) I got soundly thrashed by a passing policeman, still in his police boots and stab vest. He said afterwards that if he'd realised he was going to win so easily, he'd have kept his helmet on, 'because that would have been funnier.'

The classic sprint test – the equivalent of the ramp test, and just about the only thing you can do in a physiology lab that is even less amusing – is called a Wingate test.* You

---

* Named after the Israeli Wingate institute, in its turn named after Orde Wingate, a British Army officer who was responsible for developing modern guerilla warfare in the Far East during WW2. He was described by Winston Churchill's personal physician as 'borderline insane' and often wore a string of raw onions round his neck as a convenient snack. He also had a tendency to issue orders having freshly emerged from a shower, still naked and still scrubbing himself with a brush on a stick. Having said that, he was rather an effective soldier. There is a memorial to him in London, near the Ministry of Defence.

sprint as hard as you are able. And then you hang on as best you can for a period that might be 30 seconds to three minutes depending on exactly what you're trying to find out. The idea is that at any given point you're riding as hard as you're still capable of, so the power trace goes downwards throughout. In its longer versions it is hell – you're dying in agony the whole way. Three minutes can, I promise you, feel like for ever.

The test looks for the size of the initial 'bang', which depends on ATP and other hi-energy phosphates that are already in the muscle, and then how much you manage to hang on to, which depends on ATP being made anaerobically.

At absolute full effort, over the first few seconds, my maximum sprint best was about 1,120w. That's not quite in the so bad it's funny bit of the bell curve, but it's still very firmly at the bottom of what you'd expect for a serious bike rider my size. The hanging-on bit of it was worse – over 30 seconds my average power was only about 770w. Never mind the averages for pro bike riders, that was only about average for an active non-bike rider. Jamie's official lab-report summarised my Wingate results simply as 'terrible'.

A road sprinter like Cavendish can probably hit more than 1,500w, and could hang on to a 30-second average of over 1,000w, while at the same time being, essentially, an endurance rider. After all, he only gets to sprint at the end of perhaps five to six hours in the saddle. A pure track-sprinter like Sir Chris Hoy could probably hit 2,500w, and, again, hang on to a lot of it, maybe over 1,500w (my guess – it's not the kind of thing he went around telling people).

Sprinters are different from people like me. They've got more anaerobic ability. They can produce a great deal of energy without oxygen. There is a lot more there when they jump off the start line of a track race. In a ramp test, when they get to VO_2 max, they've got more left to give.

The quid pro quo is that they have less aerobic ability – they get to the VO_2 max point a lot sooner, and OBLA a lot sooner. The net result is that they can't ride fast for extended periods, like a time trial, but they can blitz out huge amounts of power for very short periods, like the first lap of a team sprint or the last lap of a keirin race.

It's not a whole different physiology – we're all on a continuum from people like me to people like Hoy – it's a difference of emphasis. It's in the muscles. All muscles, or rather all muscle fibres, are not the same. There are types. Endurance diesels like me have a relatively high proportion of type 1.* Type 1 fibres are excellent at generating aerobic energy for very sustained periods. They're fuel efficient, they contract relatively slowly, are resistant to fatigue, and have a high density of capillary blood vessels.

Type 2 … well, it gets a little more complicated. We actually have type 2a, 2x, and 2b, and yes, in that order.** These tend towards sprint-type characteristics. In order, each variety is progressively faster to contract than the one before, quicker to fatigue, produces higher forces, and has lower capillary density. The different varieties are actually reasonably disparate – type 2a fibres are used in exercise of up to about 30 minutes, 2x five or so, and 2b for less than a minute.

It's not strictly relevant, but muscle fibre-types are why birds like turkeys have different colours of meat – the brown leg-meat is (more or less) type 1, and the white breast meat is type 2. This is why turkeys fly in a short-term burst of vigorous, if somewhat ineffective, flapping, but can amble along quite happily on foot for miles.

---

* Type 1 used to be called 'slow-twitch', which was usefully descriptive and had a hint of poetry. Physiologists don't stand for that kind of thing, hence the change.
** They discovered a and b first, and only later found there was one that had to go in between. It could have been worse – they could have called it 2c.

There is almost no 'pure' sprinting in bike racing. The first lap of a team sprint, typically 17 seconds or so from a standing start, is probably the closest there is, using mainly a mix of stored ATP and ATP made anaerobically. By the time the effort is as long as the 30-second race for man two in the team sprint, a third of the energy is produced aerobically. A flat-out 90-second effort is around 50/50 anaerobic/aerobic. Efforts that don't go from a standing start, as for a road sprinter, or even for a match sprinter doing a qualifying 200m ride from a two-lap wind-up, have a greater aerobic component again, because the residual ATP in the muscles is likely to have been already exhausted.

Different athletes have a different mixture of fibres, and it's this that substantially determines what they're good at. Track sprinters lean very much towards type 2b; road time triallists and climbers more towards type 1. Yet even within a given event there can be a lot of variation in how the metabolisms of different individuals produce the energy required. When I was riding 4,000m individual pursuit events over four-and-a-half minutes, I was probably doing them 95% aerobically, because that was all I had. Often as not I'd be racing someone doing it only 70% aerobically – and probably training entirely differently from me.

Road sprinters are among the most complicated and diverse of all. Road sprinting is physiologically quite complex – I saw a power file from one of Cavendish's finishes a couple of years ago, and it was a long way from the steady, steady, steady, boom! profile you might expect. The final burst was relatively modest, but in the couple of kilometres preceding it there were several repeated high-intensity efforts to maintain position in the bunch, jump through gaps, and close on to the right wheels, interspersed with brief periods of partial recovery, and all of it following five hours of riding.

There is still a basic question that I haven't answered. That is, what actually stops you? In something like a ramp test, or a sprint, or in chasing an attack up a hill, what causes that horrible, helpless empty-legged feeling?

It's easier to say what it isn't, which is the TV commentator's favourite explanation for the last-lap creep, the rider's rising levels of lactate or lactic acid.* ('And his muscles are filling up with lactic acid! The finish line can't come soon enough!')

It really only has that reputation because it was one of the first chemicals that physiologists worked out how to measure. Consequently, the high levels of lactate that accompanied hard exercise got the blame for more or less everything, from causing muscle contraction, to stopping muscle contraction, to causing fatigue, as well as cramps and stitch, not to mention making your legs hurt for days afterwards. (The theory with the latter was that it formed crystals in the muscles that tore at the fibres. The main problem with it is that the sort of exercise that produces the most severe soreness is very long, very moderate aerobic stuff like marathon running or long distance triathlons, where lactate levels stay very low. The soreness is more likely to be caused by microscopic damage to the muscle fibres themselves.)

Lactate is more interesting than that. It's produced in muscles all the time, from rest upwards, in proportion to the intensity of exercise. Far from being a waste product,

---

* 'Lactic acid' is often used in armchair-sport-land as a synonym for lactate – it's not entirely the same thing, and we're more likely to be dealing with lactate as sodium-lactate rather than the acidic form. Doesn't make a lot of difference, but it's something else to shout at the television.

it's a source of energy. It's used with great enthusiasm by several of the internal organs, including the heart, and especially the brain.

It's used by the skeletal muscles too. At low intensity levels, the lactate that's produced is used there and then, which is why lactate levels stay fairly low when you're just jogging along. At higher intensity levels, above lactate threshold, more lactate gets made by the exercising muscle than it can use. It's still useful. The picturesquely named 'lactate-shuttle' uses it to transfer carbohydrate supplies from non-exercising muscle via the bloodstream, like air-to-air refuelling. Lactate is what means you can use the energy reserves in your whole body, not just your legs. In the later stages of something like an Ironman triathlon, where the effort is consistently quite high for hours on end, half the energy is typically supplied via lactate metabolism.

All this means that lactate disappears as fast as it's produced, until you get to the OBLA point – hence that point's other name: maximum lactate steady state. Go beyond that in intensity, and lactate starts to increase, even for a consistent level of effort. With a certain inevitability, better athletes are better at the whole lactate thing. Most obviously, the OBLA point occurs later, and at a higher intensity, as the lactate that's produced is used more effectively.

OBLA is a vital landmark in aerobic physiology because it clearly delimits what you can sustain and what you can't. The high lactate concentration is still not in itself the main reason you come gasping to a halt, though. That is something that's altogether more difficult to pin down. Just how difficult is shown when, as I did, you start trying to find out. I asked my long-term coach Jamie, who muttered something about calcium, potassium, and 'running out of energy', then changed the subject. Another physiologist just said it was 'complicated', then changed the subject. One of the leading textbooks, in the course of over a thousand closely typed A4 pages, contains six somewhat tentative paragraphs around about page 400, then changes the subject.

I'm not sure whether it's because of the 'lactic acid' myth, or just something intuitive from the way you feel in the dying moments of a sprint effort, but it's hard to escape the feeling that muscle fatigue ought to be something simple. 'Too much X is produced, which causes Y to stop working because of Z, and you grind to a pathetic, agonised halt.' The reality is a bit unsatisfying – it feels like a mess of bits and pieces, and as you watch your competitors vanish into the distance you're left with nothing very specific to blame.

There are several points where fatigue affects the muscle's ability to keep doing what you want it to. The increased acidity level in the muscle itself caused by lack of oxygen is the first thing you get pointed towards. There are biochemical issues, like reduced enzyme activity, that limit the amount of ATP that can be produced. And there are alterations in the levels of the chemicals that govern the ability of ATP to cause muscular contraction.

Further upstream, there are significant changes in the nervous system that controls the muscle – essentially the neurons become less effective at firing muscle contractions. And at a further remove, there are chemical changes in the brain that limit what you're prepared to put your body through. Ironically, given that we're talking about exhaustion, the list is not exhaustive. To make it even less tidy, different things seem to cause fatigue to different muscles at different times.

The most recent thinking on fatigue and failure has seen an emphasis on the central nervous system. Physiologist and distance runner Tim Noakes, who wrote the magisterially comprehensive *Lore of Running*, has suggested the idea of a 'central governor'. The thrust of this is that it's not what happens in or around the muscle that creates the feeling of fatigue and the eventual failure, but a subconscious control mechanism designed to protect the heart and the brain from damage through lack of oxygen. When the governor detects oxygen levels dropping towards a point that it deems a risk, it acts to close down exercising muscles to reduce the load to something safe, and to generate the feeling of heavy-legged wretchedness we all know so well.

This involves the slightly spooky idea of a subconscious process that's capable of predicting what's going to happen next. Your brain being smarter than you is not the sort of thing that makes psychologists especially happy. But it could resolve a lot of the uncertainties and complications of the more conventional attempts to explain the whole area. It's rapidly moving towards becoming the accepted orthodoxy.

Of course, if you explain this to any sort of halfway serious athlete, they say, 'So sort of like a fuse, then?' Followed almost immediately by, 'How do you override it?' Certainly that's what I said. Speaking as someone who came awfully close to burning his school down while manning the lights during a school play by overriding a 13-amp fuse with a nail, I should have been able to resist asking this, but the idea that there was more in there and it was only me that wouldn't let me have it was too much to bear.

It seems very likely that different people's governors will intervene at different points, meaning that the only difference between two physiologically identical riders might just be when the governor kicks in. It's not just about what you've got – the pumps and the pipes – it's about how hard you can use it. It starts to look like a whole new area. 'It's probably the future of performance physiology,' was Jamie's view, although he then added, 'even if no one really understands it.'

That's not quite true. There are some things that the central governor theory has started to make sense of. Take one of the lesser-heralded effects of EPO as an example. Aside from the changes to blood composition that it can produce in the medium term, EPO also seems to be able to increase VO_2 max as an acute response – not by altering the basic physiology, but by altering how much of that basic capacity you can use.

EPO is a naturally occurring hormone, not just a drug, and is produced as a response to altitude exposure. So, in theory at least, a blast in an altitude tent shortly before a race might produce a worthwhile benefit in the form of an 'override'.

Another current possibility is ketone drinks. Ketones are produced by the body as part of the process that breaks down carbohydrate and fat – you get elevated ketone levels after fasting, or even just before breakfast in the morning. They have an effect on the chemistry of the brain, and if taken as a supplementary drink, appear to have a similar effect to EPO in increasing the proportion of your physical ability you can actually use. Doubtless physiologists all over the world are busy working on other, related bits of chicanery.

This has been a rough snapshot of what makes up the most fundamental differences between athletes. The bad, the good and the unbelievable. It's been a static picture, taken in a laboratory, and hasn't looked beyond where an athlete is physiologically at a given point. It is the mechanics of what they can do at any given moment in time, that's all. I haven't looked at all at how they came to have those characteristics in the first place. In reality, all athletes, at whatever level, are in a constant state of flux. Life as an athlete is a process, not an unchanging state of being. That's true not just from week to week or month to month, but even from minute to minute and hour to hour within a single day's riding.

I've used a car analogy before. Essentially what this chapter did was explain how the engine works, how different engines do the job slightly differently, and how a racing engine differs from the one you have in a Ford Mondeo. All I've really done is open the bonnet and point at things. I haven't really starting dealing with how you build it or maintain it, or even what happens when you start it up and fuel courses through it to bring it to life. How it responds to the real world of training and racing. That is where we're going next.

CHAPTER 3

1,400 calories an hour: fuelling an athlete

To strip the sport down to its bare essentials, cycling consists of only three raw ingredients: oxygen, food, and bicycles. It is not hard to get riders interested in the first and last. Oxygen, more accurately, the ability to move it, is what separates the great from the good and the good from the rest. It's what defines and motivates almost all endurance-related training.

Bicycles are the world's greatest invention, objects of beauty, works of art, the tools of the trade. Most cyclists' initial attraction to the sport has at least something to do with bikes themselves, and this is something that never leaves them. Even if you incline towards the brutally utilitarian, they can provide an obvious edge over the opposition.

Food is more complicated. To be blunt, no one formed a passion for cycling because they were excited by sports nutrition. Everyone eats anyway – it's not immediately a part of sport, it's a part of normal life. Some riders, even some very good riders, more or less ignore it. Some get obsessed with weird fads. Some get hung up on vitamins, minerals, and other supplements rather than actual food. Some manage to get it about right, although as often as not that's just luck. But unlike your aerobic capacity, or your muscle fibre-typing, or your ambition, your diet is unlikely to define your career.

Attitudes can tell you something about the athlete, though. During the Tour of Britain race in 2012, I spent a day with the team helpers from one of the leading British domestic outfits. I was writing a piece for their sports-nutrition sponsor, so mostly I was interested in what the riders were getting to eat. At the end of a stage, each of them got a bag with a protein and carbohydrate recovery drink, an energy bar, and a can of Coke. 'The problem,' said one of the helpers, 'is we can give them the recovery drink, which provides exactly what they need, in exactly the right quantity, and exactly when they need it, but they'll only drink Coke. Most of the time we get the recovery drink back untouched.'

I could sympathise. When you get off your bike after a long stage you want to let go for a few moments, to eat or drink what you feel like. It's comforting in a world where comfort is hard to come by. But there is a window of about 40 minutes immediately after exercise where the body is hungry for nutrients, and will absorb them much more effectively than it will at any other point in the day. If you want to have riders capable of going out the following day and racing hard again, you have to use that window. If you don't, you give everyone who does a head start for the next stage.

A few months later I interviewed Nigel Mitchell, nutritionist for Team Sky. I asked him how the team reconciled getting riders to eat and drink what they needed post-race with their own rather more sugary instincts. 'Simple,' said Mitchell, 'we ban soft drinks. We're not pissing about, investing in all the things we do, and then handing out Coke. We're a performance team, and the riders know that. One can of Coke here or there might not hurt that much, but it's what it represents. You can't send out a mixed message.'

While the gains offered by getting nutrition right are relatively small, the closer to the limits of performance you get, the more important they become. In some ways it's the ultimate detail, the best expression of what a marginal gain can look like. As with everything else, elite riders and teams take care over details that would be a waste of time and money for even most decent club athletes.

In the interests of full disclosure, as a bike rider I was, and am, terrible at this whole area. The only reason I've never succumbed to some sort of eating disorder is that there have always been so many to choose from and I couldn't decide which one I liked best. It's telling that I learned more, and changed what I do more, in the course of researching this chapter than I did with the rest of the book put together.

It's not that I spent a career trying to support my training on a diet of Pot Noodle, quite the opposite. It's just that I never saw an eating fad I didn't like. This was not a good thing to combine with a tendency towards the obsessive. It didn't help that sports nutrition appeared to constantly change its advice. When I was a lightweight rower at university, before I switched to cycling in my early twenties, the team nutritional advice was to avoid fat and eat carbohydrate, supplemented with about a gram of protein per kilo of body weight. Total kcalories not to exceed 1,500 per day, which was a challenge when we were training for four to five hours.

I lived off small quantities of toast and low-fat hot chocolate for a term. I lost 6kg in five weeks. I also lost the ability to get to lectures and back without having to rest on every bench and garden wall I passed and wait for the dizzy spells to go away. The advice today would be significantly different: a lot more protein, a more rational mix of fat and carbohydrate, and more attention to exactly what fats and what carbohydrates to eat and exactly when to eat them. As far as we were concerned then, there was no nutritional difference between wholegrain rice and wine gums. In these modern times you'd also be encouraged to eat enough to avoid the dizzy spells that most of us took as a sign of our commitment to the cause.

As a hangover from that, for years my diet was much too carbohydrate heavy – half the world's wheat farmers are still driving tractors I paid for. But the problem wasn't just what I was eating, it was how much. Because I'd mastered the art of losing weight, I spent a couple of rather limp seasons trying to race at 68kg, rather than the 73kg I later came to settle on. Even after the carbohydrate years, I sometimes spent months trying to live off fruit, or chicken, or chicken and fruit, or some similar bit of stupidity, because I'd read a scientific paper and decided that doing this would improve some minor aspect of my physiology, while ignoring the damage it was doing to half a dozen others. As far as food was concerned, for most of my career I was an unbalanced danger, if not to my health, certainly to my fitness.

From a purely athletic point of view there are only three reasons to eat. One is to provide the energy to ride your bike, in racing or training. The second is to provide what you need to recover from long hard riding so that you can get up and do it again the next day – this is especially the case in long stage races, where calorie expenditures can top 7,000 a day. The third is to help your body adapt to the training. This is all fairly simple – it's just fuel, fuel, and building blocks. These three requirements aren't even all that hard to reconcile to each other. Every sports nutritionist

I've ever spoken to has at some point used the word 'simple' to describe what they do, albeit often as a preamble to a lecture on gene expression. I can only assume it's athletes who make it complicated.

The energy – the ATP – to ride a bike is made from food, mostly by combining it with oxygen. The rate of energy expenditure during cycling is the subject of all sorts of estimates, pored over by riders trying to lose weight, but it's generally around the 40–50kcal per mile, or 25–30 per km mark.

The late nineteenth-century experiments that first looked at rates of energy expenditure were aimed at establishing the conservation of energy, by comparing the energy input (food) with the energy expended. To measure the expenditure, they used a hellish device called a human calorimeter – a sealed, insulated chamber with an oxygen supply, a filter for removing carbon dioxide and moisture, a thermometer for measuring energy expended in the form of heat, and a poor bastard of a test subject who might spend up to 13 days in there. Some of the experiments involved cycling continuously for 16 hours, with total energy expenditures of upwards of 10,000kcal. The energy going through the bike was used to light a bulb, which can only have underlined to the subject the ludicrous position he'd been put in. (The conservation of energy was, indeed, demonstrated, and to an impressive 0.2% accuracy, which will doubtless have been a great comfort to him.)

The practical upshot was a fairly close estimate of aerobic energy expenditure, around 5kcal per litre of oxygen used. Using that, at the time trial pace I can sustain for an hour or so I'd use about 23kcal a minute, for a total over the hour of about 1,400kcal. This is a pretty ferocious way to burn through the body's reserves.

★★★

I imagine everyone knows there are three sources of energy in food: carbohydrate, fat and protein. Given the complex nature of human physiology, it will probably be no surprise to learn that they get turned into cycling in different ways, at different rates, and in proportions that change depending on what kind of riding you're doing and how long you've been doing it for.

Carbohydrate is the one we all associate with riding. Fast, available energy, easy to consume on the move, easy to use. This is any sugar – glucose, fructose, sucrose, lactose, maltose – and starch, which is how sugars are stored by plants, in large, complex linkages. When it's eaten, this can be turned into glucose and used more or less immediately, or into glycogen, which is the form in which the body stores carbohydrate in the muscles and the liver, or converted into fat.

Typically an athlete can store about 400–500g of glycogen depending a bit on body size, with 4kcal of energy in each gram, for a total energy content of 1,600–2,000kcal. When you bear in mind a rider like me can tear through 1,400kcal in a single flat-out hour, you start to get some clues about how critical the details of all this might be.

Fat is a complicated issue – saturated, mono-unsaturated, poly-unsaturated, cholesterol of good and bad varieties, all of which produces a fever of excitement in diet books and advertising campaigns, and almost all of which I'm going to ignore.

From a cycling-specific point of view, the first thing to say about fat is that as a means of storing energy, it is outstanding. 9kcal per gram means it's twice as energy dense as carbohydrate. But it's even better than that. In practical terms it's more like nine times, because every gram of carbohydrate is stored along with almost three of water, while a gram of fat is stored as just a gram of fat. It's a much lighter, more concentrated form of energy.

It can be used readily. At rest, 90% of the energy you use comes from fat. And you can store buckets of the stuff – if you ignore one or two misguided experiments, my body-fat percentage in my decent seasons varied between about 6% and 9%. That's a store of around 65,000kcal, or over 1,300 miles even at full time-trial tilt. Compared with carbohydrate stores, which are good for about 30 miles, it's an almost inexhaustible fuel tank, even on a relatively lean, medium-sized man.

Protein is not primarily a fuel source, but a small amount of it still gets used that way. For decades the assumption was that protein use in exercise was almost zero, because it was measured by analysing urine for the nitrogen that's released when protein is broken down. It turns out that most of the nitrogen is actually removed in sweat. At rest, something like 5% of your energy needs come from protein. Under some circumstances, significant muscle protein can end up being used for energy. This is not good news – it's the equivalent of eating your own legs.

As I've mentioned above, at rest, or during very easy bike riding, most of the energy comes from fat. And how simple life would be if that stayed the case as you worked harder. The problem is that not only can carbohydrate be turned into ATP twice as fast as fat or protein, it produces more ATP per litre of oxygen. So as the exercise gets harder and the energy demands go up, the proportion of energy that comes from carbohydrate also goes up.* For trained but

---

* At my first couple of lab sessions I couldn't figure out how these proportions were calculated – it sounded like something requiring blood sampling. In fact, you work out the proportions of fat and carbohydrate being burned by analysing expired air – the nutrients are metabolised with a slightly different amount of oxygen, so the ratio of carbon dioxide expired to oxygen consumed depends on the mix.

non-elite riders, at a very easy pace something like 90% of energy is from fat. By the time they get to a moderate training pace – somewhere just below lactate threshold – it's only 50%. When they get to OBLA sort of pace – the kind of thing you can hang on to for an hour – it's down to probably 25%. And finally, at the very top end, anaerobic metabolism can't be powered by fat at all. If you spend three days feeding a track sprinter a diet that only contains 5% carbohydrate, you'll render them almost useless.

The practical upshot of this is that, given the limited supplies of carbohydrate you've got, the faster you're riding, the smaller the fuel tank. I can only assume this is nature's idea of a joke.

There is another variable at work, which to some small extent mitigates this injustice. At a perfectly consistent moderate pace, the longer you ride for, the greater a proportion of energy comes from fat. This was established in 1934, in one of the all-time classic exercise physiology experiments. It involved monitoring carbohydrate and fat use over a six-hour exercise period. Initially, 20% of the energy was from fat. Over the course of six hours of continuous cycling, at exactly the same intensity, it increased to over 80%.

Unfortunately this clawback doesn't help as much as you would hope. Fat use goes up, yes, but mainly because a lot of the carbohydrate store has been used. The bottom line is that the proportion of carbohydrate being used at any point is related to how much is available. When the hammer goes down in the last couple of hours of a long race, there is still every chance that the carbohydrate tank will be empty.

In the end, despite the vast reservoir of fat available to all of us, it's still carbohydrate that is key. Elite riders aren't interested in covering huge distances at a nice easy pace, they're interested in racing, and that means that at some point, perhaps a great many points, they're going to have to go at things like they mean it. And they definitely need to mean it at the end. Whatever they do, they have to be careful with their carbohydrate supplies. The need to use energy only when it's absolutely necessary determines the tactics of almost every long race.

Running out of carbohydrate, really running out, is not something anyone looks back at fondly – and almost everyone involved remotely seriously in endurance sport has done it at some point. I used to occasionally ride 12-hour time trials – a simple, somewhat anachronistic event where you just see how far you can ride, on the road, in 12 hours. I wasn't very good at them – not only am I metabolically fairly inefficient at the best of times, but I have a tendency to burn a higher proportion of carb to fat than most riders. This combination means that really long events are fraught with hazard. In the first 12-hour I rode, I imploded after about five hours. This was the bonk, the knock, hitting the wall, in French (always adds a touch of class to your cycling) *la fringale*, but no number of synonyms were any comfort when, very suddenly, I was empty.

My vision clouded over. I felt dizzy and breathless. The classic description of what happens to your legs is that they 'pedal in squares', and I don't think I can improve on that. There was an overwhelming weakness. All I could think about was a marathon-running friend who had breezed through 20 miles of the previous year's London race in a couple of minutes less than two hours, heading for an outstanding time of about 2.35, when disaster struck. It took him well over an hour to cover the remaining six miles. He reported stumbling straight down the middle of the road because the only thing he could see was the white line, while elite runners ran past going more than twice as fast. 'I got so confused, at one point I became convinced I was running backwards,' he said. He could hear perplexed spectators wondering aloud what the old man, who'd bought all the proper running kit but clearly had never run a step in his life before, was doing getting in the way.

I had laughed and laughed at this. In the midst of my 12-hour disaster it was only the thought of my cruel, unfeeling laughter coming back with interest that prevented me from lying down in a ditch to pray for death. I'm not exaggerating. That is what a real bonk – for some reason I always think of it as a 'bonk-royale' – can do to you. It's just awful. And if it's bad on the flat, think what it's like if you're trying to ride uphill.

All the same, normally you don't go with a bang, it's closer to fading away. As blood glucose levels fall, you recede back to an increasing reliance on the slower-burning fat. The 'bangs' only come when you try to ignore this, and completely over-commit to an unsustainable pace. It's not a coincidence that big bangs rarely happen to people training on their own – part of the scenario is normally other, stronger riders, pushing you beyond what you can really do. I'd say falling for it is a rookie error if it wasn't for the fact I did exactly the same thing in the next 12-hour I rode.

It certainly doesn't help that even the process that metabolises fat to release energy is powered by carbohydrate: fat burns in a carbohydrate flame. Your body can make glucose from protein, and when you get to the furthest edge of carbohydrate exhaustion, it will do more and more of this to keep the fat flame burning. This is bad enough in a race, but if you dig yourself a hole like this in training it's a disaster, since you'll be tearing down the very muscle that you're supposed to be nurturing.

All of this rests on the basic metabolic injustice that while you can convert carbohydrate into fat, and protein into fat, and even protein into carbohydrate, you can't convert fat into carbohydrate.

The sole item of good carbohydrate news is that you can put it back fairly easily. Its availability is very closely related to its intake – and an experienced rider keeps it coming, in a nice constant stream. You can absorb about 60–80g of carbohydrate an hour. Sadly this number isn't amenable to being trained, it's pretty much fixed, and it's more or less universal. There's no point in trying to pack any more in, because over the course of several hours of racing, it will have very unhappy digestive effects.

It's not all that hard to do this. Nigel Mitchell described how they do it at Sky: 'It's simple. Everything we give them has 25g of carbohydrate in it. A gel is 25g, a rice cake is 25g, a half energy-bar is 25g, a 500ml bottle of drink is 25g. All we ask the riders to do is make sure they have three, or maybe four things an hour, as well as a bottle of water. We tried working out much more sophisticated strategies – exactly what to eat and when – but in practice it depends how the race develops. Generally they eat solid food in the early stages, or when the going is more relaxed, and gels when it's going hard. The rice cakes are the best race food we have – carb, a bit of protein, and ours are fairly moist, so there's some liquid as well.'

If you do the maths, you find you still have a problem. An elite rider can burn through anything up to 1,600kcal in a really hard hour. Even if half of that is from fat – and at that pace it's almost certainly quite a bit less – that's still 200g of carbohydrate vanishing. A steadier hour of pace setting at the front of a bunch might still be 1,300kcal, and 150g of carbohydrate. You can't put it in fast enough to ride like that all day. In a hard six-hour stage, when a rider's total calorie burn might be 7,000kcal, no matter how diligently you eat you're still always in danger of it all going wrong. This applies no matter how stellar you might be. I met Bradley Wiggins' coach, Shane Sutton, on the morning of one of the crucial mountain stages at the 2012 Tour. 'How's it looking?' I asked.

'It'll be fine as long as they make him keep eating,' he said. 'That's all that matters today.'

You can try to pack more carbohydrate in by using different sugars – adding fruit sugar, fructose, to the mix helps a little, because it can be absorbed via a different mechanism. For long time trials, and even some of my harder, longer training rides, I've tried mixing two parts standard maltodextrin energy drink with one part fructose, boosting the total hourly input to between 90g and 100g. But it's a less-than-safe strategy – you need a durable digestive system to cope with it. It's a risk you can take for single long days. For riders in stage races, whose bodies are already under a lot of stress, the knock-on consequences of a bad day's digesting could be serious.

Carbohydrate loading is the most widely known way round the limited supply of carbohydrate. It's not complicated – you just eat an awful lot of carbohydrate during the two to three days before an event. The 'classic' loading method requires you to prepare for this by purging the carbohydrate you already have – in the few days before the eating commences, you reduce the amount of it you consume and go for a few long, undernourished rides with the express aim of bonking.* This is deeply, deeply unpleasant. The more moderate method just includes the eating phase. All you have to do is consume something like 600g of carbohydrate a day for three days. This is a lot less fun than it sounds.

---

* 'Bonking' as an expression never stops being comical, no matter how often you've heard it. On a related point, there is a bike-clothing company that makes 'Windstopper Trousers'. That's going to be funny for ever as well.

Carbo-loading is common among marathon runners and long-distance triathletes, but it's very rare in pro bike riding. It's not something you can do regularly and the long days on the bike are routine for the pros. It makes weight management difficult. And, most importantly, for some reason it doesn't really seem to work very well for a typical road race with its constant variations of pace.

In the UK, where there's still a tradition of long time trials, it's used by bike riders a bit more often, and it certainly seems to work for those. But remember what I said about carbohydrate storage: three grams of water per gram of carb. Loading will hike your carb fuel tank from 400g to perhaps more than 800g, plus all that water. You end up reporting to the starter feeling like a slightly nauseous waterbed. At least if it's a hot day, all that water comes in handy for making sweat.

You can eat carbohydrate. You can even eat a lot of carbohydrate. But that's not all you can do. You can try to avoid using the carbohydrate you have in the first place. An old Ironman triathlon trick is medium-chain triglycerides, a variety of fat that consists of a shorter chain of carbon atoms than most common long-chain fats. These are absorbed via a different route from other fats, get transported very quickly to the muscle, and are metabolised very rapidly. That's the theory anyway. Some studies have shown a small increase in the pace a rider can sustain at the end of a long ride – others have shown no difference at all. MCTs are also outstanding for causing stomach cramps and diarrhoea. They're most easily found in coconut oil, or as an ingredient in some energy bars. As with fructose, it's something I've used fairly frequently in long time trials or training rides, generally with no problems. (Although unfortunately I do mean 'generally'…)

But the biggest difference you can make isn't what or how you eat. It's what or how you use it. It doesn't take a

Nobel Prize-winning physiologist to spot that if you can find a way to use more fat, you'll use less carbohydrate. Endurance training increases the amount of fat used at any given sub-maximal effort level – in fact it can more than double it.

This is why professional bike riders spend their winters packing in the long rides. Five, six, seven hours of grinding, tapping, rolling, or trundling, depending on the outlook of the rider in question. Usually done from home, even by the stars, because the off season is really the only chance an elite rider gets to stay in one place for more than a few nights, and to see their family. For riders based in northern Europe, that often means being on a bike for almost all the hours of winter daylight. The long rides shift the rider firmly into a zone where fat burning is the main fuel source, and the muscles and the enzymes adapt to it.

It's easy to assume that the long rides aren't necessary – it's not all that hard to get a lot of the aerobic adaptations in the oxygen-moving system from relatively short training sessions. But if you ask a pro who has to race for five or six hours in a day why they still, very traditionally, go and grind out the miles, their answer is simply that that is how they stop themselves from falling apart at the end of a long event.

That doesn't mean people like me haven't gone looking for a shortcut. I'm particularly keen to find one for two reasons: I've never been great at the fat-burning game, and these days, as I retreat from full-time riding, I just don't have the time. The idea of a fasted ride is an old one – get up, skip breakfast, put plain water in your bottle, and crank out three or four hours. You try to do it at a pace that doesn't involve bonking, but if you're a powerful rider with a high energy-turnover, you fail quite a lot of the time. This does help with the fat-burning adaptation, because as with the pros' long rides, you're in fat-burning territory for quite a long time. The problem is that you're quite probably in protein-burning, eating-your-own-legs territory as well. The same dangers apply to the alternative strategy of stringing together several days of long rides and little carbohydrate.

The current attempt to square this circle is to fuel the three- or four-hour ride using a mix of protein and a small amount of carbohydrate, and maybe some coconut oil, in an attempt to keep yourself in an anabolic state (building muscle) rather than a catabolic one (tearing it down) while keeping carbohydrate availability low. The protein hopefully means that even if your body starts to demand significant amounts of that as a fuel, at least it's not using muscle. The carbohydrate and the coconut oil should stave off the bonk-royale. It's not a pleasant session – you feel like you're hovering on the edge of the abyss for most of it. At least it seems to sort of work, if the lab scores are anything to go by, but it's not as good as the proper long stuff.

If the first part of the nutritional game is preserving carbohydrate while you're riding, the second part is putting it back afterwards. This isn't especially complex. You eat. You eat, and you make sure you do at least some of it in the crucial 40-minute window immediately after you finish riding. You do that because you can take advantage of a large post-exercise spike in insulin levels, which can double the effectiveness with which muscle glycogen is replaced. It works best when you combine carbohydrate with some protein. Since you probably need some water as well, a recovery drink is the most common solution

This isn't all that hard to do in training, where you're in control of everything. I remember overhearing a GB junior squad coach at the end of a training session issuing the splendid-sounding order, 'Commence recovery procedure', which just meant 'take out your recovery drink and drink it' but with a bit of added *Thunderbirds*. Most detailed recovery procedures will also specify modest carbohydrate intake every 20–30 minutes for the subsequent couple of hours as well.

At a race it can be harder, especially for those who do well. Podium ceremonies, press conferences, dope control, and any number of other things are organised for the convenience of everyone except the bike riders. But they need to use the window immediately post race, especially in stage races where the ability to recover from day-to-day is the most important part of the whole scenario.

Stage race recovery has changed a bit over recent seasons. It's not that long since most riders were under pressure to try to eat enough carbohydrate to replace all the energy that had been used – so that might be 9,000kcal on a big mountain stage. By the time they'd been on a bike for seven hours, been taken to the hotel, had a shower and a massage, they were left with an almost unimaginable quantity of food to try to deal with in the time available – most of it probably wheat-based as well, which hardly did much to help.

The misconception there was fairly simple – a lot of the 9,000kcals were fat, and there's not usually any especially urgent need to replace that. Nigel Mitchell said he's pushed riders towards quality rather than quantity. 'Even if there might be 9,000kcal being used on some stages, we probably only go for an intake of 5,000kcal, maybe even less. If you can keep a rider's gut healthy, there is a better chance they can use all of it.'

The demands of recovery overlap substantially with the third reason to eat, to promote adaptation. This is an area of rather more mystery than eating during or after racing or training. The basic objective of an athlete's life is to train and create a training stimulus. For a long time whenever I did one of my occasional training talks for a club or a coaching group, I used the analogy of your muscles containing lots of little workmen. The idea of training, I would say, was to cause enough stimulus (effectively microscopic muscle damage) to prompt the workmen to not only fix the damage, but to reinforce the repair against future damage.

As a metaphor, I thought it wasn't bad. For instance, you need to pitch the stimulus at a level which gets the little men working, but which doesn't cause carnage on a scale that they can't cope with. But eventually someone told me I sounded like a patronising parody of a primary school teacher, so I stopped explaining it this way, and took to punishing future audiences with lots of unpatronising biochemistry that I didn't understand myself. The demand for talks dried up, and the problem solved itself.

If I still used the metaphor, nutrition for adaptation is about giving the little workmen the material to work with. There is no point in training and creating the stimulus if the stimulus doesn't lead to an improvement in fitness. And there is no point in training for hours a day, over months and years, looking under every physiological dustbin in every physiological alleyway for every scrap you can find if the building blocks to turn the stimulus into improvement aren't available.

Where this differs from other critical areas – oxygen transport, bike design – is that it's all a bit less clear-cut. The experimental data is not as plentiful, or as helpful. The loads that elite riders put on their bodies are extreme, so experiments and experience that relate to more normal people can't be relied on. Elite riders are in much too short supply, and are much too expensive to maintain, to start organising realistic experiments on them. You have to begin somewhere else.

For example, before Team Sky and Team GB, Nigel Mitchell was an NHS nutritionist. He carried a lot across to sport from experience treating cancer and HIV patients. 'Gut health is the key to it. Patients – and riders – with poor gut health don't get the nutrients they need from the food. In the NHS I'd see patients with very acid guts caused by medication. If we could alkalise the gut, they'd absorb a lot more nutrients. If you bring that across to cycling, you get the same result. For years, sports doctors insisted that you needed to inject vitamins and minerals into elite cyclists because it's impossible to get enough from food. Then the authorities introduced a needle-ban, and suddenly food was the only way. That gave us an advantage, because we'd been doing it like that anyway.'

The example he gave me of how they try to manage gut pH and nutrients was vegetable juice. The team have their own chef – Søren Kristiansen. 'Søren will probably make 20 litres of vegetable juice a day – someone like Brad Wiggins probably gets through a couple of litres on his own.' Riders were struggling with the volume of vegetables and salads they were being given. Juicing it takes out the bulk of the insoluble fibre, leaving just the nutrients and the soluble fibre, and managing the pH of the gut. I knew he wasn't kidding about the quantities – one of the Team Sky press conferences at the 2012 Tour was held in the dining room of their hotel. As the assembled hacks were leaving, the waiting staff were bringing jugs and jugs of juices to the table.

'I'm interested in the effects of drugs, and what they do,' said Mitchell. 'It's biochemistry, the same area as nutrition. Something like a steroid, in endurance cycling, is about enhancing recovery. And my take on it is that you only need to use something like that to enhance recovery if you haven't got the basics of gut health right.'

Part of the gut-health battle surrounds protein, which makes the gut more acid. The first sports nutrition book I bought, in the late nineties, suggested that for endurance athletes a gram of protein per kilo of body weight per day was 'ample'. Protein recommendations have been going up and up for the entire duration of my career. Mitchell reckoned his riders eat between two and two-and-a-half grams per kilo. 'At an evening meal 60g would be fairly common – they'll have the chicken and the fish and maybe the chicken again. Then they start the following morning with a protein-based breakfast – usually an omelette.' An alkaline gut in the face of that lot takes quite a lot of work.

The biggest problem with making all this work for riders is that it's psychologically a long way from bike riding. The connection between training and going faster, a lighter bike and going faster, even a relaxed mental state and going faster is a lot more immediate. Riders who would go nuts if they missed a training session or were forced to race a bike with a dirty chain will happily skip meals and eat or drink things that they know they shouldn't. I've known several elite riders who underpinned hours of detailed, committed training a day with a diet that would have embarrassed an eight-year-old trapped overnight in a sweet shop. Once, as I was diligently drinking a recovery drink after a race, one of them told me not to be so daft. The best thing, he said, about being a cyclist was that you could, 'eat any crap you like.' He produced half-a-pound of Dairy Milk and a litre bottle of Coke from his bag and set to work. (This was a man who would have been one of the most successful bike riders in the world if he hadn't been such an utter shambles as a human being.)

It's one of the areas where team management makes a real difference – if they put riders in the position where the path of least resistance is to do it right, they get better athletes. Get the team leaders to do it right, and the younger riders coming in will want to fit in. Then you make it easy by providing food that's tempting and delivers the nutrients you want. You crack the occasional whip when you have to. As with everything else, resources help. Top teams have their own chefs. Lesser teams have to rely on persuading the hotel chef to cook something vaguely suitable. Crappy teams have to just hope for the best. Individuals left to their own care can probably be relied upon almost absolutely to get it all wrong one way or another.

Different types of rider are looking for slightly different things – for most track sprinters or BMX riders it's just about eating enough. 'The problems are when they miss an eating opportunity, especially the youngsters. Skip three or four meals a week, and they just don't develop as well as they ought to,' said Mitchell.

For endurance riders, a lot of it is about body composition – essentially balancing power against weight, and body fat against muscle. When I say 'a lot of it', for many I mean almost all of it. Body weight in cycling is an utter obsession – not just your own, but other people's as well. I've even heard rumours of pros going training with a bit of padding under their jerseys to give false comfort to their opponents, who could be relied upon to study the resulting 'spy' photos with the unhinged fervour of a *Daily Mail* picture editor.

It is a trade-off, though. Power-to-weight can be improved by reducing weight, or increasing power. Any weight-loss strategy will inevitably end up costing power – and for elite riders it will happen sooner rather than later. There comes a point where the power lost is more significant than the weight lost, and the ratio starts to go up again.

What doubles the complication is that power-to-weight only counts going uphill – on a flat time trial, the ratio that counts is power-to-aerodynamic drag. That ratio doesn't have much of a trade-off at all; the two elements are almost independent. In practice, flat riding is all about power, and weight matters barely at all. That makes two different scenarios to reconcile, and what you want depends on the characteristics of the race you're trying to win, the composition of your team, and even the competition against whom you're trying to win it.

This is without even looking at the dynamics of the training phase, where trying to lose weight is normally felt to be at odds with trying to train hard. Each of these factors would be difficult enough to navigate on their own. Together they're a maze.

For an athlete, the basics of losing weight are not complicated. You eat less, train more, or both. The amounts of energy are so large, both going out and coming in, that creating a big enough calorie deficit to lose weight isn't difficult, at least not if you're the sort of person who had the commitment to be a serious athlete in the first place. If you're training for several hours a day, it wouldn't even be that hard to run a deficit that was greater than the total suggested intake for a sedentary person.

That sort of deficit wouldn't work that well from any perspective other than raw weight loss, because the quality of your training would fall apart. The difficulty with this area is how you lose fat and build muscle at the same time. Not for the first time in our conversation, Mitchell assured me that this is actually very simple. 'You need to keep in a negative energy balance, while sustaining a sort of "micro-anabolic" state. It's about protein again: 20g of good protein per main meal, and another 20g in between and before bed.' Good protein? 'Milk is as good as anything, though we use a protein supplement as well. Then you carefully map out the carbohydrate intake around racing and training.'

Very simple, in this instance, seems to mean tracking the energy expenditure of a rider, as well as estimating the proportions of that coming from carbohydrate and fat (presumably by reference to lab results) and then feeding in the right carbohydrate quantities at exactly the right times to keep the fuel tank full enough for quality riding, but not so full that anything slops over the side and gets turned into fat.

I'd say it was a piece of cake, were it not for the suspicion that if you type 'cake' into one of Mitchell's spreadsheets an alarm goes off.

What's clear is that most of good nutrition, even in elite sport, is about getting a few basics right, and about managing the logistics so that you can do that consistently, day in, day out, to try to support everything else. 'Simple' doesn't really do justice to the amount of effort that has to go into it if it's to be done right. But it's a marginal gain that is very closely tied to a handful of fundamental principles, none of which are all that difficult to grasp.

It's mainly in order to make this straightforward world more complicated that sports nutrition has turned for years to the dark art of supplements. This area is the cause of more arguments, preaching, soul-searching and even occasionally scientific research than the rest of nutrition put together.

I'm not sure there's an official definition, but roughly, the word 'supplement' covers anything you eat that would raise eyebrows if you served it at a dinner party, and which is taken with the intention of making you ride a bike faster but which isn't a banned drug. They're almost invariably a food extract of some sort, in a concentrated form. Vitamin tablets would be the more normal end of the spectrum. The other end? Well, I suspect there's almost nothing that someone somewhere hasn't convinced themselves is a legal rocket-fuel, so the other end could be more or less anything. I've heard of coffee-flavoured yoghurt mixed with Red Bull and a spoonful of sodium bicarbonate, but I'm sure there is plenty that's weirder.

The arguments surrounding supplements are two-fold. Some argue that you shouldn't take anything artificial, anything that's not normal food. Even Team Sky's vegetable juice could fall foul of this approach, depending on just what level of a ham-sandwich fundamentalist is putting it forward. The concern is that using something artificial – although it might not itself be against the rules – could be the start of a slippery slope. Carrot juice leads to blood doping in much the same way as drinking tea often leads to a crack habit. Yet even the militants usually let their eyes slip over energy drinks, gels, and bars, which are at least as artificial as a vitamin tablet, and, if you take a broad view of what the general population takes, probably considerably more so.

The second argument points out the danger of supplements being contaminated with illegal drugs, possibly from different products made in the same factory.

When it comes down to it, almost every athlete I've ever discussed it with uses supplements of one sort or another. Some just cover themselves against potential shortfalls with a couple of vitamins. Some need considerably more reassurance – Tour de France winner Alberto Contador's submission to the Court of Arbitration for Sport at a hearing in 2011 referred to 27 different supplements in regular use.

Most athletes use them because there is evidence that most of them make some marginal difference, at least under some circumstances. Clean athletes use them because they're looking for whatever legal advantage they can find to compete with the cheats, and tend to be fairly impatient with the preaching of the fundamentalists. Paul Manning, Olympic gold medallist and coach of the women's endurance team in 2012, said, 'It's easy for the critics. Athletes these days have to be in London one week, Sydney the next, the US the next, whether they like it or not. It's not always easy to get the food you need, and if you don't get it right, you don't recover.'

If, of course, you're not a clean athlete, the ethics went out the window some time previously. No one has yet found a way of looking at cycling that makes blood-doping OK and vitamin D not.

My view has always been that a sport is defined by its rules. What you can take and what you can't are pretty clearly defined – while there are some 'grey areas' they are not all that extensive. We work to the edges of every other rule in the book, as does every other athlete in every other sport. I don't see why this one is different. If you don't like something that's legal, your problem isn't usually with who is doing it, but with the rules.

What supplements people use and how much difference they make is a whole new issue. Vitamins and minerals are, as they are for most people with a decent diet, really an insurance policy. Anything excess to requirements is just excreted – the traditional snarky joke is that the more expensive your vitamin pills, the more expensive your urine. But if something gets scraped off the pills on the way through, it's probably money well spent.

Other things tend to have their origins in biochemistry. There are quite literally dozens of them, perhaps even hundreds. While, psychologically, normal eating feels far removed from performance, the idea that there might be something special out there that's both magical and legal is deeply alluring. You could fill a book with them, and several authors have, even though supplement fashions change so quickly that it would be out of date almost the moment it was published. I've picked out a couple that are being heavily used at the moment, chosen because they're fairly representative of the way these things work/are supposed to work/con the gullible (delete as you prefer).

One supplement that almost everyone I asked said they used was beta-alanine. It's an amino acid that you can find in, for instance, turkey. It's a precursor of carnosine, a substance found in the muscles. Beta-alanine supplementation over several weeks can almost double carnosine levels. The role of carnosine in exercising muscle is a bit more of a mystery. Its most likely function is to improve the homoeostasis of the working muscle cells. But however it works, there's good empirical evidence that the increase in carnosine improves performance in high-intensity exercise – most effectively in sprint events. As an odd side effect, it makes you tingle all over if you take too much of it.

While the use of beta-alanine seems to be almost universal among elite riders, Nigel Mitchell was less sure about its effectiveness. He suggested that it wasn't much help to sprinters, 'though they all take it, probably because they like the tingling effect.' He suggested it was most useful for endurance riders who do interval training, because it would make the training efforts more bearable.

I've used it for years, based on a combination of the theory and the feeling that I've managed to spot benefits among the day-to-day and week-to-week cycles of fatigue and adaptation. I'm probably only 70% sure I'm right, but when I look at all the other tiny gains I go chasing, that's more than enough. I'd imagine that most of its other users are working on the same basis.

Beta-alanine has been around for several years now. A more recent source of interest is beetroot juice. This manages to be simultaneously both normal and odd. It's normal enough to buy in a supermarket, but, well, it's beetroot juice. In fact, it's the high concentration of nitrates in beetroot juice that has aroused so much interest. In 2009, researchers in Exeter suggested that the nitrate in beetroot juice caused both an acute increase in the diameter of blood vessels, which lowers blood pressure, and a reduction in the oxygen cost of exercise at any given intensity – a reduction of somewhere in the region of 5–10%, which is pretty significant. Time-to-exhaustion increased as well. In other words, more power for the same level of effort. That's exactly what we've all been looking for all these years.

The sports world gave a delighted holler, and started drinking beetroot juice. One of the side effects is that it stains your urine pink. At a dope control after an event in 2010, almost everyone emerged from the toilet cubicle trying to hold their sample in such a way as to stop everyone else noticing its colour was somewhere on a continuum between rosé wine and fresh blood.

Whether it made everyone go faster was less clear. Certainly very few elite riders seemed to gain as much as we were all promised, but then again, if I'd found a 10% improvement in anything, the last thing on Earth I'd have done would be to start telling other riders. Studies subsequent to the first one have shown somewhat inconsistent results. The original study was with trained subjects rather than elite athletes, and more recently a consensus seems to have built up that the benefits are reduced for highly trained riders, especially those with very large cardiovascular systems. One possible explanation is that the reduction in blood pressure creates a problem for those whose physical ability depends on a very large blood flow, but it may be something else altogether. Some exercise physiologists have stopped recommending it at all for elite athletes, concerned that under some circumstances it might even reduce performance. Despite the uncertainty, there are still plenty of top riders, including a recent world time trial champion, who still use nitrate as part of the preparation for major events. Whatever the problem is, it seems that it may be a long way short of universal, even among the small demographic of the most elite cyclists.*

I chose beta-alanine and beetroot juice as examples, mainly because they're fashionable. I could have picked from any number of others, like l-carnitine, l-arginine, sodium phosphate, Gakic, creatine, or sodium bicarbonate, and the pattern would be much the same: a sound empirical underpinning, a tentative theoretical mechanism, and a lot of debate. The problem is that almost all of these things depend on each individual's response, and it's very easy for any changes to get lost in the day-to-day and race-to-race variations in a rider's form, feeling, power outputs and heart rate. Even if a controlled experiment with a subject group of one was a plausible thing to do, you can't knock off training and racing for a few weeks to do it. Like a lot of the fine-print of nutrition for an individual rather than an averaged population, it's educated guesswork.

The one thing that I am 100% sure works – and more or less everyone I've ever spoken to about it agrees – is omega-3 fatty acids, or fish oil. There are all sorts of good reasons for taking fish oil, and it's not exactly a new fad, since it has a history that goes back centuries. For an athlete, the standout benefit is that it reduces post-exercise inflammation. You suffer less muscle soreness, and recover better.

I'm not the only fan – Mitchell brought the same enthusiasm to Sky from his NHS experiences with cancer

---

* It's somewhat outside the area of this book, but at club level, several of my slower (but no less worthy) friends swear by beetroot juice or nitrate gels.

patients. Cancer cachexia is a stress-related body wastage that's not related to a calorie deficit. Omega-3 is an effective therapy. In some respects the stresses that serious athletes put on their bodies have something in common, and omega-3 has a similar effect.

This aspect of fish oil is almost in the same territory as the post-training ice-baths we were all taking a few years ago. Again, those were touted as the solution to post-training inflammation. The problem with that approach (other than the bleeding obvious 'aargh' one) was that while it reduced inflammation, in doing so it reduced the stimulus that generates adaptation to training and improvement in condition. You hurt less, but only because, to all intents and purposes, you'd trained less.* Non-steroidal anti-inflammatories have the same unwanted consequence. Happily, fish oil does not.

The downside is that quality is critical – there is a lot of very low-quality oil out there. And unfortunately quality costs.

Water tends to be bracketed with food, for obvious reasons. But its role in exercise hasn't all that much to do with the energy system, not directly. Water's role in bike riding is mainly about temperature regulation. The prime means of keeping cool is via sweat, and hard riding on a hot day can produce anything up to three litres of sweat an hour during hard efforts, and up to 12 litres a day – though much less in moderate weather. A couple of litres' worth of dehydration

---

* My favourite memory of the Commonwealth Games in 2006 was an athlete in the village who, three times a day, had her own wheelie-bin (brought from home, presumably to no small consternation at the airline baggage desk) filled with iced water, then climbed into it and stood there glumly for 20 minutes. It was funny then. Now that I know she was worse than wasting her time, it's hysterical.

starts to be a real issue. A 2% drop in body weight reduces VO_2 max by around 10%.

I've yet to come across any modern-era bike rider who feels they'd rather save the weight – but this wasn't always the case. Jacques Anquetil, a five-times winner of the Tour de France in the 1960s, famously advised minimal fluid intake.* 'Driest is fastest,' he said. He was from an era when the race rules curtailed how much riders could drink, something they often tried to circumvent by bursting into roadside cafes, grabbing as much as they could fit in their pockets, and taking off again in pursuit of the race. They even carried bottle-openers. All the same, Anquetil's maxim was taken up by many professionals through to the 1980s.

The thing about hydration is that there is a distinct paucity of secrets. You lose water and some minerals – for practical purposes almost entirely sodium – in sweat in order to keep your body temperature stable. Most of the sweat comes from the blood plasma, with all the consequences for reduced blood volume that you'd expect, like reduced stroke volume and a higher pulse – about 8bpm for every litre of sweat lost. The increase in heart rate doesn't compensate for the reduction in stroke volume, so the total cardiac output goes down.

You replace the sweat by drinking. The main problem is that only 800–1000ml of fluid empties from the stomach in an hour, there's not much you can do to increase it. It helps a little if there's a decent volume in there, but there's a limit to how much you comfortably want sloshing around. Clearly if you can sweat at three litres an hour and only put it back at one litre an hour, you have a potential

---

* Anquetil was also at the centre of one of the first classic doping scandals. In addition to that, he had a child by his stepdaughter before marrying his stepson's ex-wife. For obvious reasons, no cycling book is complete without him.

problem. This is especially the case for pro cyclists, often competing in hot conditions for several hours a day. You can try to keep track of problems by comparing the colour of your urine to a special colour-chart, which is always a conversation-starter when you do it at a motorway service station urinal.

The only solution is to keep drinking consistently, on and off the bike. If you're not drinking with food, liquid with some electrolyte (mainly sodium) content absorbs more effectively from the blood into the cells, and keeps you slightly thirsty so you can keep drinking. At Team GB and at Sky, Mitchell said they'd never really had a problem with dehydration. 'When the riders are woken, they're given a drink, we have loads of drinks on the breakfast table. Then we keep them drinking on the bike – as well as the 500ml of sports drink each hour we give them 500ml of water. And we make sure they always have drinks in the evening.'

What's the drink? 'It's just diluted pineapple juice for the most part. We got a bit tired of making it, so we've started getting it made commercially, with coconut water rather than plain water. It doesn't make a lot of difference to the drink, but coconut water is a sexy bit of nutrition at the moment, so it gets riders a little more excited about drinking.'

The one and only hydration trick I've ever come across is to hyper-hydrate before an event, using about 750ml of weak sodium citrate and sodium chloride solution. It increases blood plasma volume, which is good, but at the cost of a significant sodium intake, which is less good. It's certainly not something you'd want to do frequently, and it's not often used in cycling. I've used it in a handful of long time-trials, but outside the UK that kind of event is a rarity. I nicked the idea from triathlon, where that type of sustained effort is more common, and where the difficulties presented by drinking while swimming mean that the extra fluid is even more valuable.

Because hyper-hydration increases plasma volume, you can, of course, use it in parallel with something like beetroot juice that acts to dilate the blood vessels. It ought, under those circumstances, to keep blood pressure up. In other words, bigger pipes and more blood to squirt through them. But it would be hard to tolerate on a daily basis, and it's exactly the kind of too-clever-by-half mucking about that goes wrong more often than it goes right.

As I said at the start of the chapter, nutrition is the world of elite cycling, and the culture of marginal gains, in microcosm. Everything else, from training to psychology to technology, works the same way. For a methodical team, coach or rider, there is a classic progression from the obvious to the obscure that gathers up smaller and smaller benefits. The decision you have to make about when you give up is, as ever, determined by the resources of money and energy you can summon up. There will always be more, somewhere.

What is different about nutrition is that there is a greater tendency for attention to slip from getting the basics right towards the more esoteric. Getting your carbohydrate intake right before, during, and after training will make more difference to your riding than any number of supplements. You would never, never know this from a conversation with a lot of elite riders, coaches and even sports scientists, who continually scout around the far reaches of the literature in search of something new.

It's not hard to understand where this comes from – in a world of detail, complication, and bringing huge resources to bear on the ideal chain lubricant, the idea that a key to performance might be a tomato and mozzarella salad applied at just the right moment seems almost absurd, not to mention very, very boring. I can only assume it's because food is so mundane and everyday that it gets taken for granted. But it's well worth getting right. I say that as someone who got it wrong for an entire career.

CHAPTER 4

3.49.999:
perfecting an athlete

I CONDUCTED QUITE A FEW OF THE RESEARCH INTERVIEWS for this book in the Manchester Velodrome cafe. It's one of the relatively small number of cafes in which you can look up from your notes and your coffee, notice that the next table has been occupied by six people who own ten Olympic gold medals between them, and think nothing of it.

I interviewed Dan Hunt there. At that point he was the coach of the men's team-pursuit squad. Previously he'd run the women's endurance programme for the 2008 Games. We were talking about the details. 'I'll show you something,' he said. He riffled through a few pictures on his phone, then handed it over. 'It's the whiteboard with the plan for London on it. It sits in my living room.'

The board was covered in numbers, at the top left the biggest one was '3.49.999', with a red box around it. 'That's the target time. We decided back in 2008 that winning in London was going to need a time below 3'50". So having decided that, we worked out what it would take to do it. You need the first half-lap in 12.5 seconds. Then consistent 14-second laps. To do that, the man on the front, if he's an 80kg rider with a drag factor of 0.23, needs 686w at 130rpm on a 110-inch gear.'

The board then showed the exact power required for the second, third and fourth riders to sit in the slipstream. Man two and man three needed about a third less power than man one. For man four, on the back, the power was actually a little higher than for the two riders ahead, because when you ride very close together at very high speeds you get a slight benefit from having someone behind you, who effectively reduces the size of your wake.

The board showed the starting efforts needed for man one to make his 12.5s half-lap – 1,700w – then man two needed 1,500w to make it there in the string one bike length behind him, man three needed 1,300w, and man four 1,200w. Even 1,200w is a massive starting effort for an 'endurance' athlete – in the days when I rode team pursuit I wouldn't have had a prayer of making it on to the back of the string. I'd only have been good for about man eight, if there was such a thing.

There were notes about the torque required off the start line: 'We brought in some of the sprint coaches to help with the peak power training to get the first few pedal revs right. Bear in mind they have to do this on a 110-inch gear.' 110-inches is only a little smaller than the biggest gear on most road bikes. Humping that off the standing start without falling over would be enough for most people. Even if they managed that, they'd almost certainly still be going too slowly by the first curve to stick to the banking. To ride it from 0–65kph in 12.5 seconds is almost unbelievable.

The board had more numbers, this time about the changes, when man one peels off and drops to the back. 'We've changed the way we ride the event. We've gone from man one doing one and a quarter laps off the start to one and three-quarters. That hurts, but it protects the three other guys. Man two does two laps, man three does one and a half, man four does one and a half. The four riders aren't equal, so we have to burn them at different rates, and we need lap-and-a-halfs to let man one recover from the start.

'We've cut down from traditional one-lap efforts, because the extra half for each increases the amount of recovery time in the string – instead of three laps they get four and a half. That's an extra 21 seconds of recovery for an extra seven seconds of effort. Also, every change costs a tenth of a second, because you lose a bike length when the front rider drops to the back. So we gain six-tenths by having six changes fewer overall.' He knew the power numbers the riders would need to do to get six-tenths back by riding faster but changing more often, he knew the lab-test results for all the riders in terms of what they can sustain for how long and how often, he had run the various options on the track, and, for this particular quartet of riders, this was the optimum strategy.

'We've got a database of every single half-lap the guys have ridden as a team, every single delivery, in races or in training, since 2008,' Hunt said. 'It's vast, it's macro'd, and we use it all the time, for feeding back to the riders, for selection. I could show you hours and hours of video of changes, guys crossing the same spot on the same boards every single time, and, critically, how the changes are affected by fatigue. High-performance coaching in the modern era has an awful lot do to with managing and navigating around huge databases of information. It's not about a pen and a pad any more.'

With different riders, the critical numbers will change, and the strategy will change, just as it did with the changing team between Beijing and London, when Paul Manning and Bradley Wiggins left the event. Another of the coaches told me that Wiggins was probably only the fourth choice for the event in 2008, despite his individual pursuit pedigree, because the team event has slid towards more and more of a sprint-type race. He only made the team because his endurance base meant he could stabilise the team in the later stages of the race, and maintain some longer turns, which meant everyone else could do their jobs better. If you want an idea of how team pursuit state-of-the-art has moved on, you need only think about an event where Wiggins was 'a bit of a diesel'.

As Hunt explained all this, I found I was looking around at riders on neighbouring tables as they ate lunch, talking and laughing. They looked like a very normal bunch. If you hadn't known who they were, you wouldn't have thought these were people who lived in a world that was arranged, down to the last detail, to make them able to do things that were extraordinary. 'We've got some good riders,' said Dan, seeing me look around. 'But none of them are superhuman. We're just doing our best with them.'

Training is simple. You apply a stimulus of some sort, and the stimulus causes your body to adapt. That much is fairly obvious. Coaching as a profession probably started in the Stone Age, when some sort of dweeby Neolithic me was told that if he ever wanted to be any good at chucking a spear, maybe he should go and practise chucking a spear, preferably a long way from civilisation.

The fundamental principle is specificity. You need to do what you want to be good at, because the adaptation matches the stimulus. If you want anaerobic power for sprinting, you apply a sprint-training stimulus. If you want aerobic ability, you apply an aerobic stimulus, and you apply it to the same muscles that you're planning to use for your desired performance.

While a lot of aerobic ability is related to the heart and lungs, there is still a great deal that's specific to the muscle

– swimming fitness doesn't translate terribly well to riding a bike, for example. If you were peculiar enough to set about an endurance cycling programme using only one leg, the performance gains would be several times greater for the trained leg than the untrained one, and the difference between the legs is that the muscle in the trained leg extracts more oxygen from the blood.

One of the points Hunt made in relation to his team pursuit riders was that they all rode low-profile time-trial bikes in all the training they did, on road or track, because it more accurately replicates the position they race in and engages exactly the same muscles. It's a simple way to increase specificity. When I was involved with the GB system ten years earlier, 80% of the training was still on standard drop-bar road bikes. The change of training bike now seems an obvious one to have made, but it still went against decades of cycling tradition.

The idea of specificity can push you in some unexpected directions. There is, for instance, some evidence that it applies to time of day. If you train at a particular time, that's when the eventual performance level is at its highest. There have been examples of swimmers who've re-arranged training times to prepare for major events where the finals had been moved to the mornings to suit TV schedules. I haven't yet heard of anyone following this up in the world of cycling. It's probably just a matter of time.

Training is able to change a huge number of physiological characteristics. Some things change a lot, some by much less, but almost everything that limits your ability to produce movement gets at least a little bit better. It's easy to take the idea of adaptation for granted – everyone knows about it and they have done from a very early age – but the way you can alter basic aspects of your own physiology is actually pretty astonishing.

The first changes are in the cells and enzymes of the muscles, which alter dramatically within just a few days to increase the muscles' ability to make ATP, and reduce the amount of lactate produced. The ability to metabolise fat increases at sub-maximal exercise levels, and the speed with which carbohydrate can be used increases at maximal levels.

Next, there are changes to the muscle fibres. Muscle-fibre types seem not to switch from one type to another, at least not very much. What happens instead is that the fibre types you train get bigger. Endurance training gives you bigger type-1 (slow-twitch) fibres; sprint training bigger type-2 (fast-twitch). With the increase in size comes more power, and more specialisation.

It has to be said that the degree to which this produces a significant increase in muscle size is a bit inconsistent. Many sprinters gain a lot of bulk, but some don't. On the other side of the physiology coin, the majority of endurance athletes don't develop significant muscle mass. But again, there are exceptions, like me: I've got legs like a Bulgarian weightlifter. Sir Chris Hoy once told me I'd got the biggest calves he'd ever seen, which I tend to accept as a fairly definitive analysis. It's deeply annoying, because it means my legs are as aerodynamic as elephant's-foot umbrella stands, and there is exactly damn all I can do about it.

Still in the muscles, as training progresses, the number of capillary blood vessels increases, and the size of the smaller veins and arteries increases. The various adaptations in the muscle and the increase in efficiency mean that, as you get fitter, for any given sub-maximal level of exercise the amount of blood flow required actually goes down because you can produce more power for less oxygen.

Under intense exercise, muscle will extract almost all the oxygen that the blood it receives is carrying. For endurance athletes, what sets the ultimate limits to performance is the amount of oxygen that is brought to the working muscles by the blood in the first place. With training, your body gets better at reducing the blood flow to non-exercising muscles, particularly the digestive system and kidneys, and freeing it up for other, more pressing purposes. Given the amount of blood that these organs normally get, this has a considerable effect.

Ultimately, though, what endurance riders need is more blood, better blood, and they need to pump it faster. It's not even a matter of better lung function – among athletes the transfer of oxygen from the lungs to the blood is one of the handful of things that can't really be improved upon. It's all heart and blood.*

You can, of course, change your heart and blood by training. Most of the critical differences in this area between athletes and non-athletes – heart size, stroke volume, cardiac output, blood volume, the effectiveness with which the blood vessels distribute to exercising muscle – can be at least partly influenced by training. You create an aerobic stimulus, and get adaptations to one, some, or all of these as a response.

Anaerobic cyclists – track sprinters – see different adaptations, largely confined to the muscles themselves. They see more than just the increase in type-2 fibre size and muscle bulk that you'd expect. They also have big increases in resting levels of ATP and phosphocreatine, which provide a store of instantly available energy, as well as in creatine, which is a constituent of phosphocreatine, and glycogen. Like aerobic athletes, they see an increase in metabolic enzymes, but this time the emphasis is on the anaerobic ones.

It's worth remembering that cycling has very few pure anaerobic events. Even the sprinters need considerable

---

* Sadly, my own gargantuan lung capacity isn't actually all that much benefit. Like my elephant legs, the fact that I'm essentially inflatable is perhaps even a bit of a hindrance, because it increases my size.

aerobic ability, because something like a 200m qualifier for a match-sprint competition requires the rider to wind up into the ten-second effort over a couple of laps of the track, so a cycling sprinter sees more aerobic adaptation than, say, a 100m runner or a weightlifter.

Sprint athletes have a much greater ability to generate lactate in intense exercise – partly that's from the adaptations I've just mentioned, partly it's from an apparently greater ability to tolerate the discomfort that comes from that sort of full-on anaerobic effort. Whether this is due to a true adaptation, or whether sprinters are just a little towards the 'meat-head' end of the periodic table of the cyclists, and just grit their teeth better than the rest of us, is not entirely clear.

I'm making this appear a bit too easy. There is a problem with all training. A physiologist can get a clear picture of what condition an athlete is in at any point from tracking training numbers, race results and from lab testing. In other words, what you've got. A performance analyst can produce a clear picture of the demands of the event. That's what you need. What's not really all that clear, still, is how best to get from one to the other. Despite all the effort put into it, the whole of training is still a bit of a grey area. The answer to the question, 'How do I improve x by 10%?' is never a definitive, 'Do nine repetitions of y twice a week and have a pint of milk afterwards.'

Certainly sports science has improved training by offering insights into what happens when a certain stimulus is created. Most of the data that's out there is empirical – it's shortening the odds by looking at the averages of a bigger cohort. But elite sport isn't about averages, it's about the outliers, and the variances between individual outliers mean that average solutions aren't likely to be enough. That's assuming the results transfer from a subject group that is probably club-level athletes at best. Even the more specific studies on how the mechanisms work have, for the moment, come a long way short of giving a coach a set of levers to pull. The best they've done is narrow the uncertainty a bit, prompt further questions, and nudge training ideas in general directions. It's telling that despite all the science that surrounds elite sport, the acts of training themselves haven't changed all that much in 50 years. Training an athlete is like training a dog – certain repeated actions will tend to have certain corresponding results. That's about the best you can say for it.

If you're an athlete you become inured to noticing the lack of certainty that surrounds training and its effects. That's pretty remarkable, considering the effort you put into it, the self-inflicted agonies, the weird details, and the damage it does to any hope of a normal life. On the basis that you want to go faster, you accept the unpredictability of the process, and just keep working. You can try to retain an element of detachment about it all, but in practice it's almost impossible to do so. If you're driven enough to train properly, you are almost certainly too deeply involved in what you're doing to stop and see it dispassionately from the outside.

This is why athletes have coaches: because keeping on top of everything on your own is simply too difficult. You need objectivity, which without help is next to impossible. You need knowledge, which coaches can bring with them, and you need the experience they've gained, perhaps from racing and training and building a riding career themselves, and by working with other riders over months and years.

You need a coach to manage the vast amounts of information that have become part of elite sport. While science doesn't provide a concrete road map for training, it does provide a very effective way of tracking progress, comparing details of a rider's fitness from one year to the next, and allowing coaches to broaden the base of their experience by providing more information about how more athletes work and respond. As Hunt said about his team pursuiters, the databases are huge, they're packed with cross-referencing, and they drive a large proportion of the decisions that get made.

Despite the obvious need for it, historically cycling has often been a little suspicious of proper coaching. The tendency among most riders, at all levels, was to slightly distrust coaches, and to display outright hostility to those who hadn't been top riders themselves. Even ten or 12 years ago, when the current GB squad system was getting itself up and running and in the space of a year British Cycling had moved from employing two coaches to employing something like 20, one former British pro complained that the organisation had 'more coaches than Wallace Arnold'. This was not only an excellent joke, but generally acknowledged to be a laser-guided criticism.

In that era, I used to write fairly regular magazine articles about training, because the assumption among magazine readers was that successful riders were more likely to know the secrets than coaches. At the time, most of my training was a mess of sessions culled from articles just like the ones I was writing, written by people just like me. The sessions were selected primarily for their unpleasantness and stuffed into an unrelenting weekly schedule until the days bulged at the seams. It may as well have been deliberately designed to blunt as effectively as possible whatever natural ability I'd started with. For the magazine pieces, I diligently boiled it down into concentrated bullet points of bad advice. Even now I occasionally wake in the night sweating at the amount of people's time and talent I was responsible for wasting.

But it was sincerely meant – I was wasting my own time and talent too. The problem with coaching yourself is that there is only one of you. You almost invariably find something that sort of works, gets you to a level of riding that you're prepared to consider successful (defined how you will, by results, fame or money, according to your self-belief and your ambition) and then you stick with it. You never explore the other possibilities, because too much comes to hang off whatever level of ability you've reached. Not unless you have a real breakneck urge to gamble with what you've got, and most athletes are very conservative. You need to have faith in what you're doing, and even more faith to introduce anything new. A coach you trust can provide that, and provide an objective eye as to whether it has worked.

That's still not the most pressing reason you need a coach. The biggest issue with training is that of your own body's limited resources. The instinct of most athletes is to train, and train, and train. The single most important job a coach has is to tell you to stop, to take a rest, to recover. Team GB's head coach, Shane Sutton, expressed it as, 'You can't over-train. But you can under-recover. And there are only seven days in a week.'

Back at the Sydney Olympics, one of the GB riders had his bike taken away from him, and his teammates were made to promise they wouldn't lend him theirs. The coach who was responsible for that once wrote me a training programme that featured a day described as: 'Rest day. This means abstinence from exercise. No cycling. No running. No weightlifting, rollerblading, walking or space-hopping. In other words, JUST FUCKING SIT THERE.'

You create a stimulus, which prompts an adaptation. But you adapt during the recovery periods. The more stimulus you try to generate, i.e. the harder you train, the more recovery time you need for the adaptations to take effect. As you get fitter, you can train progressively harder, but you're probably only generating the same level of stimulus, perhaps even less for older athletes with a big training history behind them. But you need the same recovery. You can push as many buttons in your training as you like, but nothing actually happens till you stop. The most basic possible training principle is that you have to alternate periods of hard training with periods of rest. You have to do this within cycles of days, weeks and months. If you keep pressing the buttons relentlessly, you don't have time to adapt before the next training stress arrives and you start to go backwards. In every possible sense.

This concept is beyond the psychological grasp of most athletes. I think every serious rider I know has been over-trained (or under-recovered) at some point. One or two of them have been that way for years at a stretch, or even for entire careers. If you're committed enough to train, you're quite certainly committed enough to over-train. It is almost impossible to shake off the certainty that it's training that makes you go faster, therefore the more of it you do, the faster you'll go. It's hardwired.

It doesn't help that there are hundreds of different training sessions around, each one of which purports to improve some physiological variable or another. It's impossible to contemplate one of these sessions without a voice saying, 'You could do with some of that. It would make you *faster*.' Whatever training you're doing, you can only think about all the other training you're not doing. And wondering if, somewhere, your rivals are somehow managing it all. Even Hoy, one of the most rational athletes of all, once attempted an utterly impossible twenty 500-metre efforts in one session, on the basis that he'd heard that it was what the Germans were doing and thought he ought to at least try it. 'I got to nine,' he said, 'and I was in bits. I think the whole thing was a wind-up.'

One of my favourite observations on training is from the running coach Franz Stampfl, who said, 'All training is principally an act of faith.' 'Faith' is exactly right: you believe in training; training is what makes you what you are. An elite athlete is almost invariably someone in a frenzy of observance. You want to do more and more.

If you're a full-time rider, you have a dangerously large amount of time in which to do more and more. There have only ever been a small handful of riders like me who made out a career as a full-time time trial specialist. But I knew of at least half a dozen during the early 2000s who tried it, who gave up work and went full-time supported by partners or parents to see if they could get the results to snare a serious sponsor. Without exception they went slower. Too much work, not enough recovery, and, in that era, a lack of willingness to look for the right coaching support.

The bottom line is that a rider can only do a certain amount, and that amount is determined by the demands of recovery. A coach hopefully has the detachment to help you work out what the priorities are in training – what do you need the most – work out what training sessions best address those requirements, and then ensure there is enough space left over for the adaptations to take effect.

If the sessions are hard, the amount of recovery needed can be surprising. When I was first involved in the GB track squad, I couldn't get over the way sprinters like Sir Chris Hoy, Jason Queally and Craig McLean trained. As an endurance rider, in a three-hour session I'd do a longish warm-up on my own on the track, gradually building up to about 50kph over ten or 15 minutes. Then maybe three or four 3km efforts, probably from a flying start, and each lasting a bit over three minutes. Then maybe five minutes behind the motorbike on the track as an 'overspeed' effort, or a team-pursuit-type effort alternating sitting behind the

bike with single laps of full-on riding. Perhaps a few standing
starts to finish, followed by a warm-down. I'd probably ride
20km in the hard bits, plus the warm-up and warm-down.

The sprinters would warm up behind the motorbike,
and even then wouldn't go to anything like as fast as I did
when I warmed up alone. They'd sit around the track
centre for half-an-hour swapping dirty jokes, before one of
them got up behind the motorbike again, rode a couple of
laps, then jumped past the bike and rode a lap flat out on
his own. Then he'd retire to the track centre for an hour or
so, before repeating the effort. He might squeeze another
one in before the end of the session, possibly followed by
one or two standing starts and a long, very slow warm-down.
The others would do the same. After what amounted to
about a kilometre of training, they'd head for home,
muttering that the gods were being unkind to them.

The difference, of course, is in the difference between
sprinters and endurance athletes. They were going deeper
than I could go, way into an anaerobic metabolism that I
just didn't have and never would. The stimulus they were
creating, and the damage they were potentially doing, was
much greater than anything I was managing. If I'd been a
sprinter, of course, I'd have diligently trained myself to a
standstill by doing too much.

Even as an endurance rider, I gave over-training my best
shot. On one of my early sessions with the GB squad, the
programme director, Peter Keen (Chris Boardman's old
coach) said I was the most exhausted-looking rider he'd
ever seen. When I reported this comment to the coach I
was working with he said, 'That's just because he didn't see
you last week.' I had no idea. I'd been on my knees for so
long I'd stopped noticing.

I was lucky – I had phenomenal powers of recovery. In
the early days of my career I did far, far too much, but I was

able to get away with it. I didn't exactly thrive – I'd have been faster on much less – but I survived. It was old-fashioned in a lot of ways. The old pros used to have training regimes that revolved round massive volumes of riding. It was accepted that there was no other way. A Tour rider from the 1980s told me that his brother, who raced as an amateur without a huge amount of success, was a faster rider. It was just that he couldn't cope with the training. At the beginning of a winter's work, the brother would be quicker. By the time 10,000 miles had been ridden, he'd be on his knees, and have to take months off to recover. In a more modern system he'd have done rather better, simply because someone would have told him to stop, to use what he seemed to have naturally, rather than to crush it below training that he couldn't recover from.

Full-on overtraining syndrome is a fairly wretched experience. It's not just a dip in motivation, or a couple of lacklustre performances. Things start to slip into persistent decline. Training sessions leave you utterly exhausted, despite the fact you couldn't even complete them properly. You ache. You're miserable. You can't sleep. You're irritable, you get a succession of colds, you pick up injuries you've never suffered from before, and even a minor scratch will take longer to heal. Of course, unless you have someone to point all this out to you, you instinctively try to solve the performance problems by training harder and turning a problem into a catastrophe.

The failure of adaptation is complicated. It involves hormonal imbalances, decreased neuromuscular function, even changes in brain chemistry that affect the central nervous system. Non-physical stresses – perhaps trying to hang on to a place in a team, or pressure to get results to placate a sponsor – can play a part. So can stresses entirely outside cycling. When I spoke to Paul Manning he said that the previous day one of his riders had rung him to say her car had broken down on the M6. 'I sorted that out for her,' he said. It was a small stress he could take off the rider.

If you catch it early, a few days or a couple of weeks off probably solves it. If you don't ... well, it can take months.

My own suspicion, based on experience, is that there is a vast wilderness, bigger than most people think, between optimum work and recovery, and the canyon of overtraining. You can do too much, spend your life too tired, but still be a decent athlete. The better your powers of recovery, the longer you can survive in it. The graph of return against outlay is a flattened bell curve. You can live on the downslope on the right-hand side for a long time. But you'd do better on less. And you could do the same on much less.

There are as many ways of doing the coach's job as there are coaches. It's tempting to draw a contrast, with traditional, old-school, flat-capped pipe-smokers at one end, and men in lab coats at the other. There was perhaps even a point in the 1990s where it was a valid dichotomy. (Though I'd also have to say that a high proportion of the men in lab coats were up to nothing admirable.) In elite coaching now, though, it would be a simplification of a process that at its best has to use both intuition and science.

Shane Sutton was the head coach of both Team GB and Team Sky during the 2012 season – he stepped back from the role with Sky at the end of that year. That puts him in overall responsibility for eight Olympic gold medals, first and second in the Tour de France, wins in three of the year's other biggest stage races, and several other things that in many other seasons might have seemed like a big deal, but which in the context of that lot amounted to loose change.

He's a former pro-rider, with a solid but not stellar career from the late 1970s till the mid-1990s.* You'd probably have put him in the old-school category. He's certainly got a traditional approach to a lot of it, and was a successful coach in the days before the British squad system really hit its hi-tech stride. On the other hand, when I suggested this view to one of his sports-science qualified colleagues, I was told simply, 'Don't worry, Shane understands the science.'

'The science', however, is not the starting point. When I asked Sutton where you start he said, 'You start by working backwards from the gold medal.' Like Dan Hunt and the whiteboard beside his TV? 'Exactly. Sometimes the basic demand of the event is very simple. Team pursuit? All you have to do is maintain the team's pace for the second half. Match sprint? Only two different kinds of ride, from the front or from the back. You take it apart from there, work out what you need, and work out what's stopping an athlete from doing it.'

Rebecca Romero was an example cited by several coaching staff. Originally a rower – she'd won an Olympic silver medal in 2004 – she then moved to cycling and went on to win the women's individual 3,000m pursuit in Beijing in 2008. 'The women's pursuit is about hitting 400w, for three and a half minutes, at a cadence of 115rpm,' said Hunt. 'When Rebecca arrived from rowing, she had big, big VO_2 max, big peak power, so the 400w and the three and a half minutes were not a problem. All she lacked was the ability to pedal fast enough – when she started she couldn't get much higher than about 95rpm. All we worked on was power-at-cadence – within a day of starting with us she was riding rollers. I know plenty of cyclists who've been riding for years who've never learned to ride rollers.'

---

* Well, not stellar by today's standards. Everyone was reasonably impressed at the time.

(Rollers are a simple indoor training method with very little resistance, which naturally leads to high-cadence riding, but they're tricky to ride.)

Sutton described the process as, 'We trained her like an elephant', which is poetic, if a touch cryptic. I took it to mean that she trained with one specific, relatively simple event in mind, and very quickly learned how to do it perfectly.

Rebecca left the programme after the individual pursuit was dropped from the 2012 Olympics. 'She wasn't a bike racer when she joined us,' said another coach, 'and to be honest she probably still wasn't when she left. But her determination to ride pursuit well was absolutely phenomenal. She beat people who, if you just looked at the simple physiology, should have beaten her easily.'

So the coaching process generally starts with something relatively intuitive. The more scientific approach backs that up. It uses data on the event and on the riders to produce real detail on what's needed and what's missing. It uses knowledge of the riders' physiology to set exact marks in training – trying to address the need to produce the maximum stimulus for the minimum of fatigue. And it monitors progress, and compares it to data for the same rider from previous seasons.

Wiggins' 2012 Tour and Olympic time trial titles were the result of a training programme designed by Sutton and Tim Kerrison. Kerrison is a former rower, with degrees in both sports science and information management, who has a background in coaching both rowing and swimming. While he was working for British Swimming he amassed a vast database on not only the GB swimmers but on the competition as well – details of every single time split, qualification rounds, breathing patterns, what side they breathed at different stages of the race. Anything that might conceivably be useful was logged, and often as not accompanied by video, so that a GB swimmer going into a race would know everything there was to know about the opposition, even if the opposition was someone they'd never even heard of.

Kerrison came to cycling with no experience of the sport at all. 'In rowing,' he said, 'the coaching is largely about technique. In swimming it's about numbers – lengths, speeds, work/rest ratios, intervals. I came to cycling curious about how it worked. In truth there wasn't a lot of either. From a coaching point of view, cycling seemed less developed as a sport. An awful lot of what pro riders do is based on tradition, and you end up scratching your head about how much of it is done that way because it's a good way to do it, or just because it's always been like that. My job is to use an applied scientific approach to coaching, to help coaches do a better job by using better science. So we had to work out what to keep, and what to throw away.'

The crucial part of the team's preparation for the 2012 Tour was a series of training camps in Tenerife. This was a change in itself – the traditional approach was that riders got fit by going racing. Racing generates plenty of loading on the riders whether they like it or not, and psychologically it's an easy way to get fit, because you just turn up, the race starts, and from then on you're led by a competitive instinct. Ten years ago, the GB team pursuiters spent their time trying to get to as many stage-races as they could to create a training overload. The plan back then was for riders to progress into major pro teams, and then have a basic diet of major events to underpin their condition. As the team pursuit grew more and more specialised, and further from the typical character-istics of a road rider, that never happened.

'The problem with just racing,' said Kerrison, 'is that you have no control. The race goes too fast, or too slow, or over terrain that's not what you need, or it's got a time trial where you'd rather have a mountain stage. You can't give riders rest days when they need them. When Bradley crashed out of the 2011 Tour, we decided he'd go for the Vuelta a España. He had a broken collarbone, so all he could do was ride the indoor trainer. He couldn't do any racing before the Vuelta at all, but we were able to address all the issues on the trainer. We could simulate almost all of what he would have been looking for from racing, but with more control.'

The training that Sutton and Kerrison talked about from the camps certainly takes its starting point from racing. 'Say we do three hours,' said Sutton, 'then we get them to do two minutes at capacity, so say that's 550w. ('Capacity' is the maximum power output a rider can sustain over five minutes in a lab test – regularly used as an endurance rider metric.) Then roll easy for three minutes, then straight into 20 minutes at threshold behind the motorbike, then finish with a 12km uphill time trial effort. It's simple, we do the capacity effort when they're fresh and can go deeper, the threshold effort recreates the latter part of a stage, and the TT is a mountain finish.'

There's certainly an intuitive underpinning there. But there is detail as well. 'The details of a session would cover an A4 page,' said Kerrison. He gave me a different session from a Tenerife camp as an example. 'A big day. Six hours, with 4,000 vertical metres of climbing – we probably do 16,000m a week. Four efforts: the first on San Miguel climb, two minutes capacity, one minute recovery. Then into 27 minutes of mid-zone three, with nine minutes at a normal cadence, nine minutes at 50rpm, and repeat.' The low cadence is to improve torque, it makes it easier to follow an attack in the mountains where the need is for a sudden acceleration against a low inertial load. Zone three is just sub-threshold (OBLA or MLSS, to be technical, but for historical reasons generally referred to by coaches as 'threshold', just to be confusing), so mid-zone three is a very little backed off from time trial pace.

'Second effort,' continued Kerrison, 'is the same, except that it is 32 minutes; ten minutes of low- to mid-zone three, then a one minute spike at five-minute capacity pace, so you get zone three, a spike, zone three, a spike. Third effort of the day, on the Grenadier climb, is low- to mid-zone three, and ten minutes of normal cadence, ten minutes of torque. Fourth effort is on a different climb again, and it's more high-zone three, but this time every two kilometres we do a sprint of progressively 15, 20 and 30 seconds.

'A lot of what we were doing with that is trying to get Brad in a position to follow an attack in the mountains at 450–500w, then be able to recover at 420w. We needed to do this, because while he can ride up a mountain at his own pace as fast as anyone, if someone with more explosive ability jumps away toward a summit finish, they could gain a few seconds. Explosive power is pretty trainable, so we broke it all down into cadences, torques and different sorts of sprint. Everything we do has a physiological justification. And it's impossible to get that sort of thing from just going racing, because you can't "train" in a race and do the efforts you want to do, when you want to do them.'

(He says that – but I remember doing a road race that included Wiggins at a circuit in West London in about 2002, where he attacked like clockwork every five minutes, rode hard for a minute or two, then sat up and drifted back to the bunch. Every time he went, half a dozen riders went after him, and were sorely disappointed when he slowed down rather than tow them to the finish. Eventually he paused for an extra minute, then went for good, and I took a lucky guess and followed him. I was sharing a coach with him at the time, which made it easier to spot. 'Tactical genius, Wiggins,' said a friend of mine afterwards. 'You never knew what he was going to do next.' I didn't have the heart to tell him that he couldn't have been more wrong. However, it would be a lot harder to do this sort of thing in a serious race.)

The target power output for each of the zones changes as you climb, because there is less oxygen available. So the same physiological points occur at different power outputs. That means if you train in a mountainous environment, the zones will be different depending what climb you're using. It will also vary according to how long the rider has been training at altitude. The climbs for each effort are picked for their gradient and their height above sea level.

The justification for altitude training that Kerrison gave me wasn't the traditional one. 'It's just getting acclimatised to racing at altitude, because the big tours are decided in the mountains, and if you just go straight to altitude you lose 7% for every 1,000m up, and the highest finishes might be 2,500m. It's not really about looking for a haematological effect.'

'Altitude tents?' I asked.

He said he wasn't sure. 'Real altitude is hypobaric – the air pressure is lower. Tents just reduce the concentration of oxygen, but at normal pressure. It's a different physiological effect. We used them a bit before and after the camps, just to try to extend the stimulus a bit, but that's all. They're not the same as altitude training.'

As you can imagine, given I've been sleeping in a tent for a decade, this cheered me up no end.

I found the level of detail a genuine shock. I'm well used to the idea of training, used to the idea that a certain workload is necessary if you're going to reach your potential. Like Kerrison, I always felt that the traditional 'miles, miles and miles' approach of pro cycling to generating this workload was pretty blunt.

Until quite recently, amateur riders had, in many ways, more sophisticated training. When I first started cycling I stole a lot of my training information and sessions from running, rowing or swimming (all sports I'd been involved in to some extent) rather than try to copy a pro approach – though that was largely because while I still had an academic job I didn't have the time to behave like a pro.

When I did start riding full-time, I kept most of the specific sessions, and added a lot of general mileage as well. I have to admit that it worked. Going from riding ten hours a week to riding 30 hours a week did make me go faster.

The irony was that when I retired as a full-time pro, I went back to something a lot more like the way I trained as an amateur, and I went faster again. Not massively so – my 40km time trial pace went up from about 400w to something more like 420w, or about one kph. The biggest average power number I ever hit was 470w in a 16km time trial in 2008 – three seasons after I'd stopped riding full-time, and in a year when my training had been heavily curtailed by the need to finish writing a book. But I was really nailing the sessions that I was doing. I can only think that the reason training for just ten hours a week worked so much better then than it had years earlier was that I'd got a lot better at actually doing the sessions – my skills as an athlete had improved.

It seemed likely that there was some way of combining the benefits of the traditional and the specific. If, for instance, I'd ridden a big winter of steady work, then a spring with more detailed sessions worked in? Or included more specific work in the long springtime rides, rather than rely on a fairly steady (traditional) pace? It was one of the things that prompted me to start asking the questions that led to this book.

But I didn't expect the precision or the focus that I kept finding as I went around asking questions of current elite coaches. They always described what they were doing as simple, or obvious. And in a way it is. The knowledge is there, the technology is there, the commitment is there, so why wouldn't you do it that way? The idea that the approach is somehow novel is very hard to hang on to in the face of it appearing so right.

Where the game comes back from the science towards something more intuitive is how you actually get riders to do all this: 'Hey, guys, we're all going to go and live at the top of a mountain for a month. There's going to be no internet, no phone reception, you're going to be away from your families and friends, and there will be nothing to do except ride really, really hard for hours every day while I drive behind yelling at you; you'll eat food selected for its nutrients rather than its taste, and you'll sit about getting bored. Oh, and we'll have a couple of media and sponsor days where a whole pile of people you'll hate on sight will ask you the same stupid questions over and over again. Who's in?'

A coach needs to get a rider to buy into what they're doing, to enjoy training, and the environment in which they do it. It's part of the process. As Hunt put it, 'One happy day every four years isn't enough, because what they do is so hard. Riders need to be told what the plan is. Why they're doing what they're doing, what the expected gains are, what the physiological justification for it is, and how it relates to the actual event.'

There is an art to this because the explanations will change from rider to rider, depending on their own view of what they do and how they motivate themselves. Personally, I like detail. If a coach wants to talk enzymes and gene expression, that keeps me interested. A lot of riders like something that feels a bit more intuitive. A small handful just want to be told what to do.

There is more coaching art in the sessions. There is more than one way to press most physiological buttons. Hunt said of his team pursuiters, 'You need imagination to give certain physical loads to different people. Some of them will happily set about a long effort – several minutes in duration. Some of them will really struggle with it, they'd rather hit shorter efforts, and more of them, which the guy who likes the long stuff can't take. There is a psychological stress to any hard session, and while you don't just want to have people only doing what they like, you have to try to make it all palatable.'

When the art of coaching combines with the science, the way riders will buy into a coach's grand plan can be quite striking. I spoke to Kerrison not long before the London Olympics. He outlined what they were doing with Mark Cavendish. Cavendish is a seriously talented rider and a hard worker. He also has a reputation for really, really not liking sports scientists with laptops.

The main problem with Cavendish winning the Olympic title was Box Hill. Not an especially terrifying climb: shortish, and not very steep. But done nine times, at race speed, it did represent a significant obstacle for a non-climbing sprinter. So, working backwards from the medal ... 'For each lap, we worked out how fast we reckoned the bunch was going to go up the hill,' said Kerrison. 'Mark can lose a few seconds on the climb and he'll still be OK, so we add that. We know the gradients on the climb, so then we know what power-to-weight he needs – and we can get that by dropping weight or increasing power or both. We know what numbers he needs for each climb, so we know what he has to be able to do to be in the bunch at the top of the ninth climb, make it back to the finish, and then sprint.'

Even on paper, this has risks: 'The problem is that if we turn him into too much of a diesel, he'll make the finish fine, but he'll have no sprint. We need to balance the diesel against the express. If we get it wrong we might even end up trying to get his power-to-weight ratio back down in order to preserve his sprint.'

At the Tour de France, a couple of weeks before the Olympics, I ran into Rod Ellingworth, Cavendish's long-standing coach. I asked him how this project was going. 'We've got him down to 69kg, which is his best weight. We've worked on the specific climbing demands of something like Box Hill. We've got his five-minute capacity up from 444w to 472w. And he's still sprinting OK. So it's all looking good.'

This is a significant redesign of an already indecently successful bike rider, all for one event. Months of work, changed training, and considerable risk to the results during the rest of the season. It was something he was prepared to do based on a sports scientist's model of the demands of a modest hill, previously notable only for the National Trust cafe at the top. Even ten years ago there is no way such a thing would have happened.

Of course, on the big day the plans all turned to spaghetti, for reasons that had largely to do with the rest of the British team being unable to control the race. But that doesn't take away from the process that led up to it. There's not much point in the analysis if you're not going to trust the conclusions. That it all went wrong, and that there was always a very substantial risk of that, just emphasises the weight that everyone was prepared to put on following the numbers. Just because something doesn't work out in the end doesn't mean it wasn't the best bet.

'If you're a scientist,' said Sutton, 'there's always a temptation to see seven days in the week, and want to put something in each test tube. It's easy to look at the numbers getting better and want to keep pushing, but in the end a training programme is just a guide, it's there to get a rider out of bed and doing something. A week before the Tour last year, I told Brad to stop training. Tim wanted him to keep working for another day or two, but I said, "He's done. We're not getting any more." A week is nothing in terms of fitness, and he needed to stop.'

Perhaps those last few days before an event are the hardest, for everyone. There is a terrible feeling of lack of control. Running down the training over the last couple of weeks, everyone has done almost all they can. It's called the 'taper'. It comes at exactly the point where you very badly want to cram, like you would for an exam. But you can't. The switch from 'training I'm going to do' to 'training I wish I'd done' is instantaneous. The internal dissonance is called 'taper-madness'.

The idea is to produce an athlete on the day who is fully rested, relaxed, and as adapted to the demands of the event as they can possibly be. Someone who is at the absolute top of their curve. The rough of it is that the volume of training comes down and the effort level stays high for the bits that remain, but it's dangerous to generalise. Individual coaches try to get individual athletes to the right spot in their own ways.

It seems blindingly obvious that you rest before an event. Yet the day before the 1912 Olympic marathon, the South African Christian Gitsham set off to run the full 26.2 miles. His coach caught up with him after 12 miles, and returned him to his hotel. Eight years later in Amsterdam the US team raced each other over the full marathon distance 11 days before the event. Tapering really only started to be taken seriously in the 1950s and 1960s. When a Dutch swimming coach introduced the radical idea of a three-week ease-up in training before the 1962 European championships, the entirely unheralded team swept all before them. The overall improvement varies widely between athletes, and between disciplines, but can be anywhere between 0.5% and 8%.

While the techniques vary, and the lengths of the taper vary from a few days to several weeks, there are solid physiological markers that they're trying to optimise. Hormones and muscle enzyme concentrations will increase as the athlete recovers, as will glycogen levels. But there are things that tend to pull the other way – for an endurance athlete, for example, there is a real need to keep blood plasma volume up at the same time as trying for complete recovery, and the easiest way to do that is by doing some short, harder efforts right up to race day.

Some coaches and athletes taper progressively all the way. Some take a block of days off completely before going back to training moderately on the last few days before competition. Many, probably most, have a serious pipe-opener in the last couple of days – for track riders this is often done as a full dress-rehearsal with all the relevant kit, diet supplementation, and warm up in place as it would be on the day. They go all the way through to the starting effort and hitting the required pace on schedule, but with the length of the ride cut back considerably.

All of this is in a pre-competition atmosphere that will be thickening all the time. There are final selection decisions to be made as the taper approaches. For an Olympic team, with a handful of places available every four years, it's never going to be easy for anyone who doesn't make it. It's even worse in a very strong team, like GB's running into the London Games, because making the team is probably harder than winning the event, and usually making the team isn't something as simple and objective as a race, it's a decision that someone has to make.

It's not easy for coaches either. I've heard of coaches in that position running trial after trial, in the hope that the decision would make itself, until eventually someone further up the management chain tells them to just bloody pick someone. The irony is that it's usually obvious who they're going to pick, they just can't bear to tell the other rider that they're not going to make it.

Inevitably, a set-up like the GB uses its huge databases. They track riders over months and years, and use the numbers to predict who's heading for the best form. Even if they're in a block of heavy training they ought to be able to tell who's likely to bounce back best through the taper by comparing previous data.

The final decisions for London 2012 were made at a pre-Games training camp at the velodrome in Newport in South Wales, where I spent a couple of days hanging about in the background. One of the more contentious issues was the women's team pursuit selection, where Wendy Houvenaghel lost out on the place to Dani King – and it was clear that there was some tension over it at the time. Houvenaghel was clearly riding strongly.

The coaches' justification for going with King came down to different types of physiology, specifically muscle fibre-types, not just performance. 'Dani's a fast-twitch [type 2] rider, Wendy much more slow-twitch. Dani's always going to see a much bigger rebound during the taper,' I was told. In other words, the more sprint-orientated a rider, the more they can expect to gain during the last days. A trial race a week or two earlier would have produced a different decision. This approach isn't always popular with riders. A lot of them, perhaps even most of them, would rather deal with something more objective, like a straight winner-takes-the-place selection race, something that's more within their control.

A curiosity of the taper is that it affects men and women differently. Women lose form much more quickly when they stop training – quite why no one seems to know. I've heard suggestions ranging from 'smaller quantities of free testosterone', to the idea that men are physiologically (and not, I was told in no uncertain terms, psychologically) able to train harder, so it takes them longer to recover, during which time they keep improving. Whatever the reason, the upshot of it is that women athletes have a shorter taper period.

For track events and time trials, even sometimes for road stages, the warm-up is the final act before the coach and the team must let go, and send the rider or team into the heat of the race to fend for themselves. The point where, whether they're ready or not, there is nothing more that can be done about it now.

The warm-up is not quite like anything else you ever do. It's not really training, and it's not really racing. It's in between. It's the transition from the athlete whose life is dominated by training and preparation and patience, to the racer. There's a totemic quality to it, which is as important as anything purely physical. Just going through the routine forms a buffer between the race and everything that went before. Forty minutes of peace, some time to think about what you're about to do during which everyone will leave you alone. When the coaches, physiologists, psychologists and performance analysts who surround a star rider or team all have to step back, the routine normality of a warm-up is a lifeline. If a rider can put on their headphones and get on the stationary trainer in the midst of a track centre, or outside the team bus at the Tour de France, and just do what they've done a hundred times before, it makes what they're about to face familiar. You can warm up and calm down.

You have to remember it's a physiological transition as well. You need to do it right, because you need to set your body up for something that can be horrifically demanding. You need to switch your body's systems on, so that you can use all the ability you have right from the race start.

It has little to do with getting warm. Warmth does increase the firing speed of muscle a little, especially sprinters' muscle, but there's no benefit to going beyond normal exercising temperature. At the 2012 Olympics, the GB sprinters used 'hot pants' – to all intents a pair of shorts made from an electric blanket – after the warm-up. It was just a way of preventing a damp, sweaty rider from suffering too much of a drop in temperature while they waited for their event.

Most warm-ups are trying to do relatively simple things. An easy spin to start stimulates fat burning, increases blood flow, and dilates blood vessels. A build-up of intensity into a few harder efforts starts to stockpile enzymes and stimulate hormones. For an endurance athlete, part of the idea is to ease the transition into full-on effort. Aerobic metabolism always takes a little time to catch up with the energy demands after a standing start, and in the meantime the job has to be done anaerobically. If the warm-up can stimulate aerobic enzymes, it reduces the lag and preserves some of your anaerobic ability for later in the event. How hard you can finish a race might depend on the warm-up you did an hour before.

Warming up matters more for sprinters than endurance athletes. Not only are the short explosive events the kind of thing you badly want a chance to mentally prepare for, the enzymes and hormones that drive anaerobic metabolism can be more significantly influenced than their aerobic counterparts. The risk of fatiguing type 2 fibres means that sprinters warm up for longer, but generally at a very easy pace, with just a handful of very short, very hard efforts of maybe just a few pedal revolutions.

I've done my warm-up under an armed guard in a portable toilet block in India. I've done it amid chaos at a Paralympic cycling event in Italy, where the team only managed to find the tandem I was riding with a visually impaired partner a few minutes before our start time. I've done it during a tropical downpour in Australia. The warm-up insulates you from all of the surroundings. It tunes you into a level of excitement. It's always the same, and that sort of stability is what any rider always wants. It reminds me that however complicated I might often manage to make it feel, bike racing itself is a very simple thing to do. It's a good thing to think about as you roll to a start line.

CHAPTER 5

A rider like a robot: the psychology of an athlete

I HAD SUCH HIGH HOPES FOR SPORTS PSYCHOLOGY. LONG ago, prompted by the confident assertion of a top professional (I forget which one) that '90% of time trial ability is in the mind', I decided to train my brain. It was probably raining outside.

From the perspective of the present, the statement has all the plausibility of a claim that 90% of chess-playing is in the pancreas. It was at best stupidity, at worst an attempt to deflect attention from all the other things going on in the late 1990s that might more realistically have been reckoned to constitute 90% of time trial ability.

In my defence, everyone thought then that psychology was the key to all the riches sport had to offer. The talk was of little else, and there was a perception among those of us who knew nothing about it that it was the shortest of shortcuts. In much the same way as I always buy the second cheapest bottle of wine, I bought the book with the jacket blurb that promised the second-most extravagant results, because I didn't want to be unrealistic.

On a warm, summer afternoon, I lay down on my back in a darkened bedroom, as instructed, wearing loose clothing, my arms beside me, palms downward, eyes closed, and I 'visualised'. I summoned up on a flickering screen in my head the forthcoming Commonwealth Games, an event that was clearly going to be a critical moment in my career. I knew it mattered more than everything I'd done up to that point.

The book had told me that the more detail I could include, the more effective the mental training would be, so I took in getting to the venue on the Games bus and getting changed in a tent. Since the Games were in Manchester, I visualised lashing rain. This is not a joke. I went through my warm-up at about half-speed, the better to absorb the nuances. I rolled to the start ramp, seeing every face in the expectant crowd. And then I rode the race, right there in the gloom of my bedroom.

The idea was that by rehearsing the actions – I'm afraid I'm quoting from memory here – you 'fire all the neurons involved in the action itself! This means your nervous system will already be highly trained before you even attempt the actions for real!' In other words, just add muscle.

After a bit of practice, I got pretty good. My heart rate elevated a little, my breathing got faster. It felt real. When I switched my attentions to track racing, I found that if I tried a similar exercise with a stopwatch in my hand, I could time the four-and-a-half minutes of a pursuit race almost perfectly. Had I been a bit more astute, I'd have found it significant that the time I always got on the stopwatch was the time I could already do, not the one I needed.

It didn't ultimately make me a better bike rider. It made me a considerably worse one. I quoted the book from memory because eventually I burned it; one of the only sensible things I ever did in the field of sports psychology. What I was endeavouring to do was brainwash myself into trying harder. This was understandable. The problem was that I was already trying as hard as was feasible. There wasn't an 'extra 20% of my aerobic system' that I'd never noticed knocking around in there. There never is.

What I achieved instead was to carefully and diligently wind myself up into a state of the highest possible anxiety. I'd have been nervous anyway, but by the time the Games arrived, there was almost no blood left in my adrenalin stream. There were crowds. TV cameras. Helicopters. A team official who told me I'd better deliver or I'd never ride internationally again. By the time I rolled past the expectant faces to the start ramp I had the most advanced case of the screaming heebie-jeebies ever recorded in the literature.

The race was a fiasco-royale. Instead of a skilfully sustained hour of cycling fireworks, I just chucked a match into the open box of rockets. There were four laps of a seven-mile circuit. Even if I'd only had to do one lap, my pace for the first few miles was far, far too fast. On the first time up the major climb, a fit-looking middle-aged man tried to run alongside me for a few moments, gasping impressed encouragement. By the fourth lap he was ambling along beside me, sipping tea from the lid of a Thermos, and saying things like, 'Never mind, son.' He ran out of conversation long before he ran out of breath.

I rode the course that day appreciably slower than I had in training – and bear in mind that in training the roads were open to traffic, so I lost time at every junction. My psychological preparation had knocked my pacing completely off its gimbals. Normally I'm outstanding at the subtleties of judging an effort – from the 'go' I can feel the difference between the fastest I can sustain for an hour and the fastest I can sustain for 62 minutes. It's the skill I built a career on. At Manchester 2002, I was too nervous to feel anything more subtle than a gunshot wound. I reverted to riding like a 12-year-old in his first race. I think I was about 14th, but I've never actually checked, because I can't bear to.

The aftermath of that particular balls-up saw me refer myself to a professional sports psychologist, and ask her to repair some of the damage I'd done to the inside of my own head. I spent most of my time with her colouring-in pie charts that illustrated the exact proportions in which my minor inadequacies as an athlete contributed to my total inadequacy as an athlete. I never found this as enriching an experience as I was clearly supposed to.

On the other hand, she taught me to visualise properly – to use it as a tool for improving technique for the handful of difficult motor skills that cycling demands, or for preparing myself for a stressful event by simply getting used to some of the sights and sounds. I tried it for the starting effort out of a gate in a pursuit race. This skill is harder than it looks. You have to shift your weight back, so your back side is far behind the saddle, then throw yourself forwards in the split second before the countdown reaches zero.

If you time it exactly, your weight is moving in the right direction as the gun goes and the gate releases. You're already a fraction of a metre down the track, and you can pull the bike after you. But go too soon, and your body weight is so far forward that the unweighted rear-wheel spins uselessly when the gate releases. Too late and you lose time – maybe up towards a second – or in extreme cases just flop over sideways on to the floor. Whichever, your start has turned to custard, in varying shades of embarrassment.

The psychologist made me close my eyes, and explain to her exactly how I was doing this. Then, as before, to see it. And this time, not just to see it, to do it. At this point I realised that I couldn't actually do it right in my head. In my head I was fumbling about, mistiming it, losing vital seconds. I crashed the psychologist's chair at least once. Sometimes, by hazard, I got it right, but not more often than once in five or six starts. It was a perfect facsimile of reality. The reason I couldn't do it properly was because I didn't actually know what I was supposed to be doing. I had no idea that level of incompetence was even possible.

However, in the end, the impact of this revelation was limited. First, I mentioned it to a coach at Manchester, who said, 'Christ, you don't want to see a psychologist. You know —— ——? He was pretty good until a psychologist got hold of him and turned him into the kind of idiot who can't put milk on his Weetabix without 20 minutes of existential angst.' That wasn't encouraging. Second, my area of cycling needed few of the refined motor skills that visualisation might have helped with – time trial pacing seemed a rather ephemeral thing to attempt to hold in your mind's eye. Third, the psychologist started skipping appointments, presumably because trying to help someone who struggled so badly to even imagine success was too dispiriting a prospect. So I gave up.

The big problem with psychology for someone attempting to do what I'm doing in this book is that the only athlete's head I've ever seen from the inside is my own. The difficulty is exacerbated by the fact that every athlete knows most of the right answers: I'm focused on my own performance; I try to control the controllable; I don't worry about what my competitors are doing; I'm taking it one race at a time; I just want to enjoy the competition, and be as good as I can be.

I can look back to press reports when I provided all of these answers and many more equally stultified, while simultaneously being obsessed with the performance of others. I was profoundly insecure, and trying to control things that were as much within my command as the clouds. I tend, unfairly, to assume that everyone else lies about it all as well. I have to remind myself that people who are better at the sport than I am are probably also better at controlling what's going on in their heads. I have to accept that of all the attributes of a properly top performer, the one in which I'm almost certainly most lacking is the right psychology.

Most people's grasp of psychology in sport has moved on from the one that so many of us shared in the days when I was frying my head in a darkened room with the idea that all you had to do to go faster was convince yourself that such a thing was possible. The general perception among fans and the media now is that an athlete who is able to deal with the pressure is more likely to win, and that the aim of sports psychology is simply to help them do this.

Even the new realism probably overstates things. It's most likely inherited from skill-based sports – golf, darts, cricket – where complex motor actions are learned, practised, and have to hold up under pressure. Often the specific skills involved, once perfected, occur with minimal or zero conscious input. They're dealt with substantially by the spinal cord, without ever even making it to the brain. It becomes a deeply everyday action, like running downstairs.

Disaster occurs when, let's say, a golfer under pressure suddenly, after years of worrying about the wind, the distance to the hole and whether he can carry the bunkers, but letting the bit with the golf club look after itself, starts thinking about the details of how to swing. He regresses to the golfer that he was before swinging a golf club was an automatic act, and slides all the way back to being a novice. Imagine the potential consequences of running downstairs while you concentrate on exactly how you run downstairs. It's why golf occasionally features a final round where one of the leaders' games disintegrates into something that would make a 24-handicapper look sheepish. They can forget everything, because they didn't really remember it in the first place.*

When it comes down to it in cycling, no one forgets how to do it. Famously so. You just forget how to do it well. In terms of sheer self-conscious wretchedness, my Commonwealth Games race was every bit as awful as the worst final-round collapse you can imagine. I still beat a lot of people who were suffering from no form of crisis at all. Cycling, at least in its execution, is not a complex sport. When I asked the British team's psychiatrist, Dr Steve Peters, about the relative importance of an athlete's mental strength, he said, 'You have to have the physical ability, or you're not going anywhere. Mentally, someone of average ability could maximise their potential. But they wouldn't be the next Chris Hoy.'

He did concede that someone with the ability, but a wretched mental approach would probably not get very far either, but it was clear which bit of the package mattered most. While he didn't name any names, it's not hard to think of one or two well-known bike riders from the last few years whose mental fragilities seriously undermined their physical ability – yet they still made it.

---

* There is a corresponding idea that people who learn a skill more intuitively – that is to say they work a lot of it out for themselves rather than get taught step by step – are much less prone to sudden disintegration because they haven't got the same early stages of bit-by-bit concentration to return to. The problem is that this is in almost all other respects a slower, less reliable way to learn a skill. The same issues might also explain why those who learn very young might be more durable under pressure.

The reverse wouldn't be true. You have to take it seriously – it's an advantage for the grabbing. But it's not a whole new you.

British Cycling's take on psychology has changed somewhat since I was being discouraged from having anything to do with it. The boss, Sir Dave Brailsford, is a man with a serious interest (and a degree) in sports psychology, to the extent that he's made it central to both the national and Sky teams. He pointed out something that I've been so close to for so long that I'd stopped even thinking about it, which is that sports psychology isn't just about race day. 'You have to manage your lifestyle so you can train to extreme levels,' he said. 'You organise your life round it, you do it when you don't necessarily want to, you eat the right foods, you make sure you take your coach's feedback to help you improve, you engage with the equipment issues, you get ready.

'Once you put a number on your back, that's different. That's where most of the general interest in sports psychology comes in. But cycling is so physically dependent, conditioning and training are so important, that the prior psychology makes much more difference. One of Bradley Wiggins' strengths is his compliance to the programme. When he's really engaged in what he's doing, he'll do 95% of everything the coaches ask.'

I hadn't ever looked on this sort of thing as being unusual. I'd never stopped to think about it at all. I, like most of the others who ever got anywhere, slid into that sort of lifestyle both gradually and willingly. I'd never thought of it as an issue of psychology, certainly not that the psychology of commitment might be more important than the psychology of racing. It hadn't really occurred to me that it was something a team would take seriously as an issue in its own right.

'In a lot of ways,' said Brailsford, 'Shane Sutton is a life coach. He makes people feel good about themselves. If he can manage to get 95% compliance from some of the star riders, then everything else will take care of itself.'

Sutton does indeed make people feel good about themselves. At the end of the interview I did with him, he asked me about my plans for the coming season. He jumped up to his whiteboard, and started outlining a couple of new sessions he felt I ought to try. He was talking about some pretty tough riding, but he did it with an enthusiasm that made me want to go home and get straight to it. He's also well known for a willingness to deliver the odd kick up the arse when it's needed – but I suspect he can manage a rider's psychology without having to resort to it too often.

You get involved in serious sport because you want to go faster, you want to race, you want to race better, and ultimately you want to win. But I'm not aware of a professional rider – certainly I don't think I've interviewed one – whose training life is motivated solely, or perhaps even substantially, by the thought of winning things. 'Winning' is too blunt and too unpredictable to hold in your head as you try to perfect a dozen or more things about yourself. It doesn't happen very often, either. An Olympic athlete only gets their chance on the biggest stage once every four years. A top road rider will probably target only one or two major races a year. Sir Chris Hoy put it best. He said simply, 'There isn't enough winning.'

Motivation probably isn't even the right word – serious athletes can still train, eat and live right when their motivation is at rock bottom. There is a more basic commitment to what they do.

It's not always easy to articulate how that commitment works. It's even harder for people who suffer from it. If you ask an athlete what drives them, the answer you get depends on when you ask the question. If you asked Wiggins as he stood on the Tour de France podium in Paris, you'd get a rather different answer (or at least I strongly suspect you would) from the one you'd get if you asked him in the middle of a wet, cold ride round the hills of north-west England on a Thursday in December.

Riding a bike has its own pleasures. And, if you're lucky, money is nice. But what matters is the process. I asked Hoy about his sporting abilities as he grew up. I sort of knew the answer – as a BMX rider he was ranked second in the UK, as a rower he was a silver medallist in the UK junior championships in the coxless pairs. He played rugby for his school, and his school was one that took rugby seriously. It's a more broadly based sporting hinterland than most cyclists, and I asked the question because I was curious to see if he thought he had basic genetic talent.

Instead I got a much more interesting answer: 'In every sport I did – rowing, rugby, BMX – there was a kid who was a star,' he said. 'Someone who picked it up easily, who excelled, who you thought was really going somewhere. I was second, or third. Maybe sometimes I'd win. But I always had to really work for the second or the third. The kid who looked like a star often as not chucked it in after a few years. When I was 14, 15, it was hard, because I was a small kid – I didn't grow till I was 16, and in the 14–15 age group there were six-foot guys with moustaches.'

What this helped to produce was a tendency to measure his achievements against himself and his own expectations, rather than against other people. So here is the bit to make a psychology convention stand up and cheer: 'It's not about being the best. It's about being my best.'

This is the grade A* answer. And, coming from Hoy, I'm sure it's absolutely genuine. This outlook has some fantastic consequences for the mental stability of an athlete. One is that it stops defeat from being too discouraging – I'm guessing, but my suspicion is that the stars from his youth tended to quit when they started to lose. Another is that when you do win, it stops you from being satisfied with that. If you think you can do better, you'll go right ahead and try to do better. As Dan Hunt put it, 'These guys can win Olympic gold, break the world record, do the event to the highest standard that anyone in the history of cycling has ever managed, and still come away thinking about how they can do it better next time.' Winning is one thing – keeping winning is entirely another.

Commitment, if you're that well adjusted, comes from looking for the improvements. From looking at the problems, and trying to work out how you solve them. A few seasons ago, we came to the conclusion that since the main hole in my physiological profile was that I was metabolically rather inefficient (the way I use vast quantities of oxygen and fuel to produce a great deal of noise and heat, but not, relatively speaking, all that much in the way of actual forward motion) maybe we should do something about it.

We tried long rides – a couple of five- or six-hour efforts a week for the few months of the pre- and early season. This had worked early in my career, but at the cost of leaving me too exhausted to even summon an eye-roll and a hostile glare for anyone who tried to tell me I was overtrained. The measures we put in place to prevent this happening again failed, since they amounted to 'if you feel tired, take some time off', and if spotting the bleeding obvious was going to work, it would have worked the first time.

Then we tried shorter three-hour rides, but in a partially starved state, so nothing to eat first other than a tin of tuna – almost straight protein – then a drink during the ride that was also mainly protein with just a very little carb. That had a benefit, in that it made me better at burning fat rather than carbohydrate, but it didn't really change the fundamental problem, it just changed the fuel.

Then we tried short efforts on a trainer – ten seconds on, 20 off, repeated for a couple of 20-minute blocks. Then we tried the same, but in hypoxia, which was interesting because the protocol in 13% O_2 meant that what felt like a relatively easy session while you were doing it could leave you in a daze for four hours afterwards.

None of it really worked. But in between times I didn't half get some bike riding done, and we found out some other things that we could look to for the next thing to try, the next step forward. It was exciting. This is what's called enjoying the process. Deriving your kicks, not from winning, not from competing, not from achieving any precise goal, but from exploring what you can do, what your body is capable of, looking for the ways to improve, the ways to get an edge.

That is, of course, just splendid for everyone involved. In some cases, like that of Hoy, and for me, in my later career at least, that is exactly how it works. For many, perhaps even for most, the commitment issue is a muddier puddle altogether. It's a balance, or it ought to be. In 2008 Ed Clancy, a member of the GB team pursuit squad, offered to have his collarbones broken and shortened, to improve his aerodynamics. I would criticise this ludicrous overenthusiasm for the cause, except for the fact that when I heard about it I thought, 'Great idea!' and contacted an orthopaedic surgeon, who told me I was 'nuts'. (A diagnosis I'd have had to pay more attention to if it had come from a psychiatrist, obviously.)

That's just a silly, if entirely honest, example. Most of the issues are more subtle. I'd say that, of the riders of whom I asked the question, 'How do you get yourself out the door in the morning?' a very clear majority, of endurance riders at any rate, said, 'Well, you just get on with it, don't you?' or something very like it.

The massively successful Paralympian Dame Sarah Storey said that training was just what she did, in the same way that writing was what a writer did. She was totally certain that she'd have been training whether she was ever in a position to win anything or not. It was just something she liked doing. A former world champion said they felt they were a compulsive exerciser – if they weren't in motion, cycling, running, swimming, something – then they weren't really happy. It was something they needed to do, and they'd been that way for years. They were just lucky that they'd got the basic talent, the coaching support and the intelligence to turn something between an eccentricity and a disorder into something between a virtue and a living.

That's not the only 'problem' you can turn to your advantage. 'Have you noticed,' said one rider, 'how many pro-rider tweets and blogs and the like are concerned with food?' Good point. The word 'cake' occurs almost as often as the word 'bike'. 'Most of them get through the long rides by bargaining with themselves about the cake at the cafe stop and what they'll have for dinner.' Calories out, calories in. The further you ride, the more you can eat. If you get it right you can eat like a black hole and still end up with the physiology of a hatstand. You can turn chocolate into gold.

I think there's a little truth in that, at least for some riders. Cycling is a weight-sensitive sport – the lighter you are, the faster you go, especially uphill. Early in my career, one of the best-known coaches in the UK told me I needed to lose 'at least a stone' (six or seven kilos). At the time I weighed 70kg and had about 8% body fat. Unfortunately for the drama of the current narrative, instead of this precipitating a decline into anorexia, I just decided he was a knob and ignored him. I was grown up enough to know that my trying simultaneously to weigh 63kg and race bicycles was preposterous. I could certainly bear to lose two or three pounds, but 'a stone' was just designed to cause damage.

I still played the 'another hour out here in the cold and I can have … ooh, what can I have? Maybe half a bar of Dairy Milk as a treat with my recovery drink. Then … hmmm … a roast beef sandwich. Or perhaps a rice pudding after dinner …' and so on. Not, you'll notice, a dream about four cheeseburgers and a bucket of Coke. It's a very focused sort of crazy. Was this unhealthy? I'd have said that it was just a small reward. By strict definition, it's bulimia. I used to weigh out food, calculate the calories in all my meals, and keep a diary of it. Which is at least a tiny bit screwed up, but it's no more screwed up than almost everything else I used to do. (There was a more dubious phase when I coached my marathon-running girlfriend, and weighed her food for her. I'm prepared to admit that might have crossed a line.)

As a motivational tool, it can work, especially for endurance athletes putting in the long rides. But it's clearly a bit of a high-wire act – while I'm sure there are athletes for whom it is a struggle, most of the elite performers must be managing to keep it all in a perspective that is at least no more messed up than most of their other perspectives, because a serious eating disorder would be hard to run in parallel with a serious cycling career.

For a start, the nutritional demands of the sport are just too high. Even an athlete who's losing weight has to eat, objectively speaking, a lot. More pressing, as a motivational tool the pre-emptive cake-strike will only help with the long miles. It actually militates against the harder, faster training, the brutal stuff that only lasts for a few minutes, because however hard you do it, it doesn't burn much and it leaves you too tired to go and burn anything later. To get back to the beginning, it's not just the commitment to train, it's the commitment to train right. All sorts of neuroses and compulsions might be part of that, but the athletes who succeed weave it all into something very sophisticated, something that goes almost unnoticed, even by them. The idea that psychology is what separates the best from the next best might even be true, sort of. Just not in the way most people think.

'Ideally, what we want is a rider like a robot.'

The GB track team spent the last couple of weeks before the London Olympics at a training camp at the velodrome in Newport in South Wales. With just a few days to go to the Games the riders were at the height of their powers. In a quiet, echoing velodrome, watched only by the coaches, and a solitary spectator (me) skulking in the stands, they did exactly the things that they were very shortly going to do in front of an audience of millions, the things that they were going to do to bring in gold medal after gold medal. I felt as if I'd found a secret hangar with a new stealth fighter in it.

The 'robot' comment was made by Dan Hunt. The men's team pursuit squad that he had there in Newport, training on their own in an empty track on an overcast Wednesday afternoon, were riding the event better than it had ever been ridden. All he wanted was for them to do exactly the same thing a week later. If they could keep their minds out of the Olympic Velodrome, with its cameras, the lights, the crowd, if they could not even take a glance at the notion that they'd spent four years working their way towards this moment, or what winning a home Olympic event would mean, it would be simple. All they needed to do was what they could already do, what they were doing in a big shed just off the Newport Southern Distributor Road, and it would be easy. Do it like robots.

That's what I had wrong all those years ago. For most of us the big occasions aren't about finding more, they're about hanging firmly on to what you've already got, and not letting the pressure ('This is the most important four minutes of your life: if you BALLS IT ALL UP TO HELL you'll never forgive yourself') take a wrecking-ball to the inside of your head. Normally it's not so much rising to the occasion as not drooping to the occasion.

I've already accepted that the cycling choke is not the most spectacular in sport. It's marginal – there are certainly athletes who compete successfully at the highest levels who go into competitions while in a state of mind that would render them useless in golf, tennis, or even football. But there are still skills, even if they're sometimes quite subtle, and you have to make sure you hang on to them, whatever it takes.

You will remember my ride in the 2002 Commonwealth Games, as recounted at the beginning of this chapter. Skip forward to the same event in 2006. There I carefully and deliberately persuaded myself I was in for an arse kicking. I looked up the results of the other competitors, and worked out what sort of margins of defeat I'd be dealing with. When they weren't big enough I repeated the sums till they were. On race day, since there was not the slightest point in worrying about the result, I just turned up and rode round the way I'd do at any other race. It wasn't exactly positive thinking, but it did what I wanted, in that it left me just trying to do my best. I ended up fourth, which was as good as I was capable of.

I've described this experience to several friends, rivals, even one or two heroes, and been surprised how many of them have approached at least some races the same way. It's not textbook sports psychology – indeed, none of my fellow travellers on this one were prepared to be named in public – but I'm reasonably certain that for most people it works better than getting too wound up about it.

My personal wrecking-ball was always the simple one of worrying about the result, which is why writing it off at the outset worked. There are, however, any number of things to worry about. Failing to meet expectation from fans or the media. Letting down teammates. Disappointing a family who've perhaps sacrificed a lot in their own lives for you. Technical things like descending, or judging the compromises to be made on a climb between riding at your own pace and following the attacks of others. Paranoia about other riders' doping practices and whether you're competing on a level playing field. The list is endless.

Steve Peters, the GB cycling team's psychiatrist, became something of a cult figure through the last two Olympic cycles. He helped produce a squad that seemed not just nerveless, but to be quite genuinely enjoying the challenge of producing their best on the biggest possible stage. Riders like Sir Chris Hoy and Victoria Pendleton credited him with large parts of their success. He even made considerable progress in sorting out the notoriously erratic snooker player Ronnie O'Sullivan.

When I spoke to him, I'd have to admit that the first 20 minutes of the conversation went tremendously badly. The recording is of one of those car-crash interviews, where my questions got longer and longer, and the victim's answers got shorter and shorter.

At that point he was kind enough to tell me why it was going badly, why I was asking all the wrong questions, and what I might usefully do to ensure we didn't waste another 30 minutes of both our lives till his next appointment. The experience gave me the distinct feeling he could fix more or less anything.

The main reason my interview started out so badly was that I was looking for universal solutions – preferably 'universal' solutions that 'as luck would have it' applied specifically to me. I was being an athlete, rather than a writer. I wanted Peters to say, 'Well, most athletes come to me with the problem that they're overly concerned with the result, and the pressure that they put on themselves to win.' Then I wanted him to say, 'And here are the three things you need to think about to solve this problem instantly.' Nothing is that simple.

Peters' model takes three elements of the brain – the human, the chimp, and the computer. (As one of his athletes said, 'it's a very modelly model.') The human is the rational part, the chimp is the irrational part that functions according to basic instincts, and the computer is the bit that gets on with stuff automatically. The art is for the human to recognise the anxieties and instinctive fears of the chimp, and cope with them. And ideally that leaves the computer to get on with running the show.*

'You don't want the chimp to ride the bike,' said Peters. 'The chances of success are enormously variable. Anything could happen. You don't want the human to ride the bike either, because it thinks about everything and analyses

---

* A considerable simplification. I liked Steve's book, *The Chimp Paradox*, very much, though since one of its strengths is that it avoids giving you idealised examples that would be a distraction from whatever specific hang up your own chimp has. It's not a passive read; you need to work thorough it with a certain amount of commitment.

every move. You want to use the computer. You want to do it on autopilot. People in what they call "the zone" are more likely to succeed. Sometimes they describe it as surreal – you're totally confident in yourself. Confident in what you can do. You believe you've done the work necessary to get what you want. You have no fears. You want to be there, and you want to compete. You're very calm, calm but competitive. There is flow.'

The computer 'thinks', but only by producing a pre-programmed response when it recognises a certain situation. It doesn't do anything original. Things bypass both human thought and chimpish instinct. 'You want to get an athlete to the point where imagination and interpretation are the last thing they start doing in a race.'

Not hard, then, for Peters to tell me what the outlook most likely to lead to success is. It sounds like a wonderful place. Hell, it sounds like a cloak of invincibility. How could anyone who feels like that not win? The problem is that reliably getting there, or even anywhere near there, isn't easy. The things that get in the way are too variable. They're individual to each athlete. And they're often a long way from, 'Don't be nervous, there's nothing to be nervous about …' or even, 'Just do your best.' Like everything else about cycling at the top level, it's about dismantling everything to see how it works, and seeing if it can possibly be made to work better.

While Peters isn't really a fan of specific examples, when pressed, he suggested the hypothetical one of a rider who says, 'I drift off during a race – I miss crucial breaks.' His response would be to ask the rider's coach what's happening. The coach might say that the problem is that the rider has a tendency to ride too far back in the bunch, so that he's having to work too hard among the wheels to go with the break, even supposing he can react from back there.

'Then we'd get the rider and the coach together, and I'd try to help them understand what they each wanted. Suppose,' Peters suggested, 'that the rider says he's worried about riding too near the front in case he doesn't have the legs to stay up there. He thinks that if he rides at the front he'll crack altogether at the high, sustained pace and perhaps not even finish the event. I'd ask the coach what the chances of a successful outcome are (be that a win, a medal, or whatever) from riding at the front – maybe it's "only" 50% – there is a substantial chance the rider is right. But maybe riding at the back, while making it more likely he'll finish the race more or less in one piece, means the chance of a win or a medal is now only 10%.'

All this is set out. How the rider approaches it is still up to them – Peters' contribution is, he said, neutral. He's not solving problems of his own selection, he's helping others to solve theirs. The rider might decide they're going to stick with their way, and if they can make it work results-wise, I don't suppose anyone would mind.

If they decide to do it the coach's way, however, the next question is how they're going to feel about it if they get the soggy end of the 50/50 chance and crack completely? 'I'd be bloody angry,' says the hypothetical rider. So then they work through why they'd be angry, whether that would help, and so on. It's not hard to see that if you can successfully work through the problems, the underlying reasons, the solutions, and the consequences you'll produce a very stable athlete. 'I need to deliver an athlete to the coaches in a condition where they are receptive to coaching. That's the key,' said Peters. 'You just keep working down these avenues like a flow chart and bringing in anything relevant till the rider is happy.'

It sounds so simple, but for the riders it's not. You're dealing with some pretty fundamentally rooted instincts and conditioning. You don't change your approach to a race, to your career, just because someone talks you through the logic and the probabilities. Believing at a rational level isn't enough. The mental exercises, the specific routines to help riders look at things differently aren't easy. Emma Pooley said that the mental training was much harder to do than the physical – though that didn't mean for a second that she questioned its value – and she wasn't the only one.

Pooley also said there were days when frankly she'd love to let the chimp get on with riding the bike – she said it seemed simpler. I know she was joking, but there's a hint of the huge change of outlook that's needed, if you think about how many riders use their mental quirks (the kindest of many available words) to motivate so much of what they do on a day-to-day basis.

The mental training is also something that needs to be done long before race day. Peters said he could help someone who began to choke under the pressure of competition, and probably put them back on track immediately, but only by referring back to the work they'd already done and to thought processes they had rehearsed for months. 'We'd have a plan, we'd have done it over and over, there'd be nothing new. Certainly no punching your hand and saying, "What we need to do is …"'

With someone he hadn't previously worked with? 'I could say, "It's all right, calm down," but that would be about it. Even just telling someone they're not alone can be quite reassuring, but I can't wave a wand and fix things.'

The irony that underlies most of professional sport – that winning is the thing you almost never think about – means that winners almost never think about winning until they've actually done it. Always the process of winning overshadows the winningness of winning. Hence the frequent bewilderment of victory.

A much-overlooked detail of Bradley Wiggins' Tour win in 2012 was a strategy put in place for winning – how was he going to react to the emotions and the pressure of making history? How was the team going to deal with that? At a practical level, how were they going to reconcile the demands of the press and the sponsors? And (the reason for the whole thing) how did they get him from a win at the Tour to the Olympics a week later without him losing focus?

For most who win, it's just a relief. The more you've already won, the more relief is dominant. The pure joy of victory is the most transient emotion there is. For most of those competitive enough in spirit to make a career out of something as trivial-yet-difficult as sport, the pure joy phase of their careers is probably a fading memory by the time they're old enough to vote. It tempers into feelings of achievement, then to satisfaction, and finally to a whooshing relief that they made it, that all those days, weeks and years ruled by total perfection in the utterly trivial have not been a wasted life.

Victory is not worth any less for this. But a professional sportsman crossing a finishing line in front does not feel the same way a fan does watching him.

For those who do not win, well, it's hard to know what they think, because no one really asks. The personal satisfaction of having done their best, having done something they enjoyed? Crushing disappointment? Both? It's a doubly difficult question, because while success is normally quite easily defined, failure is more nebulous. You might not be Olympic champion, but if that was even in your terms of reference, you'll have won some other stuff on the way, and it's a very big call to decide that every bike rider who doesn't win the Tour or the Olympics is a failure. Or, if you look back to the era most of my serious racing coincided with, do you classify someone who competed cleanly but at a modest level as a failure compared to Lance Armstrong? My experience (not bitter, no not at all) is that most people did, and even now, they still do.

When it comes down to it, winning is absolute, losing is not, because there's always a chance to pick yourself up and try again. By the time that ceases to be true, no one really cares all that much. You win in a blaze of glory, you lose in a fading away.

CHAPTER 6

Free speed:
the technology

IN ABOUT 1997, WHEN I WAS STILL A GRADUATE STUDENT, I bought a Lotus 110 bike frame. You'll know this better as the Chris Boardman Lotus from the 1992 Olympics – to be more precise, it was the next-generation refinement. I bought it from a man in Norwich who worked for Lotus, and who'd acquired it when a batch of the frames were returned to the firm by the Gan Pro Cycling team and sold off to staff in a coffee-break auction.

That, at any rate, is what he said. His classified ad in the back of *Cycling Weekly* asked for only £250 – which was a fraction of what the frame was worth, even second-hand. When I got to his house – about 45 minutes after buying the magazine and then driving to Norwich from Cambridge as if my hair was on fire – I found a small flaw in the frame's bottom-bracket threads. It would be a trivial repair, but it gave me an excuse to beat him down to a totally unbelievable £150. The fact the defect had never been fixed also made it clear that the frame had never even been built into a bike, so it increased rather than reduced its value. I managed to control a life-long instinct for being a smart-ass and didn't tell him this.

It was clear that driving home with a Lotus 110 frame in the boot for an outlay of £150 had involved someone being robbed. But whether he'd stolen the frame from Lotus, or I'd all but stolen it from him was not clear. I decided it must be the second option. This was on the basis that, short of a police raid while I was still drinking coffee from a Lotus mug and sitting on the sofa he'd made from some car-seats, I was going to buy the frame come what may, and at least possibility two wasn't a criminal offence.*

At that point, the frame was the most aerodynamic ever made. In fact, it's still right up there. Out of curiosity I took it to a wind tunnel last year and discovered that it was only just beaten by the best of the current crop of aero bikes. The thing was years ahead of its time.

Back in 1997, all I could see when I looked at the lovely, fluid shapes of the carbon frame was free speed. It was speed that didn't depend on being fitter or stronger or mentally more resilient or yet more pernickety about what I ate. I could feed my obsession with money rather than effort. I had no objections to effort, it's just that I couldn't see where any more of it was going to come from.

If speed is exciting, free speed is bewitching. There are some wonderfully well-adjusted riders out there who couldn't give a toss about any of it, who have the self-confidence to rely on themselves rather than some trick frame or wheel or helmet. At the season-opening Tour of the Algarve a couple of years ago one rider was presented with his new time trial bike, which he'd never seen before, never mind ridden, just before a wet and slippery prologue stage. He said he'd rather stick to his road bike. If it was all

---

* I did discover, years later, that it was all entirely straight. Lotus were already getting out of the bike game, and ended up with several frames and no official means of getting rid of them, so they did, indeed, sell them to staff for whatever they could get.

the same with the team management, he'd rather not kick off his season by crashing on an unfamiliar bike and breaking a collarbone. The coaches produced a laptop, tapped in a few numbers, hummed and hawed a bit, and announced that the TT bike would save him six seconds. The rider gave them a withering look, and used his road bike.

He was right. But if it were me, I'd still have wanted those six whole seconds much too badly. I've done all kinds of ridiculous things for much less than that. In 2010 I switched all my wheel bearings to ceramic versions, at a cost of about £800. You could hold a wheel and spin it, and it went round at what looked like the same speed for so long you gradually became convinced that it was actually speeding up. I used to amuse myself with them for hours at a time, which was just as well since I couldn't afford any other entertainment by the time I'd paid for them.

I subsequently worked out just how much it had saved me. Over a 40km time trial, calculated to a tenth of a second, it saved approximately nothing at all. Even bodging the sums furiously in the direction I wanted them to go, I could only get to about five seconds, and I knew I was kidding myself every second of the way. The problem is that bearing drag on a well looked-after bike is almost nothing to begin with. And even if you halve it, well, half of not much is still not much.

That wasn't the worst, though. In 2011, someone persuaded me that shoe insoles must make a difference, given they were a vital interface between your feet and the pedals. Within weeks, I had so many insoles I had to clear out my wheel-bearing cupboard to store them all. I never managed to work out a way of calculating how much difference they made in terms of actual speed, perhaps because it would have taken the resources of CERN to detect it.

I was right about the Lotus though. It did make me faster. Not by an unbelievable margin, but the advantage was clear if I switched back and forth between it and something more conventional. At the time I reckoned maybe 20 seconds over a ten-mile race. Or, in the language I'd use these days, 20 watts. It took me to my first national title, and the rides I did on it got me my first pro contract. It was £150 well spent. Speed at £7.50 a watt is as good as it comes. No one will ever get it that cheap again.

Most of my friends refused to believe this was possible. The bike was, they said, too heavy to be fast. In 1997, a racing bike typically weighed about nine kilos. The Lotus was more like ten. I was worried enough about it to save what weight I could with the components I used, down to a pair of plastic brakes that weighed nothing, and didn't come close to working. They didn't even press hard enough on the rims to make a squealing noise. They just gave you something to curse at as you waited to arrive at the scene of the accident. Picking weight off a bike, gram by gram, had been the obsession of racing cyclists since the 1860s. But that was all changing.

Saving weight makes intuitive sense. It makes even more when you look back to the nineteenth century at some of the ironmongery that riders were trying to haul up hill, without the benefit of gears. Above all, it appeals as a metric because it's easy to measure – show anyone a new bike, and they will all pick it up by saddle and bars, bob it up and down a little, and tell you that it's not as light as it should be for the amount you paid for it. Cyclists have been doing this routine for ever.

The thing is that weight doesn't make all that much difference, at least not in the margins we're dealing with. Up a steep hill, yes, it helps, and on a road race the steep hills are where the racing is at its most intense, so there it makes some sense. But for most of the history of cycling the weight obsession encompassed everything. When Eddy

Merckx attacked the hour record, on a pan-flat track, all the magazines were full of wonder at the lightness of his bike. It gained him practically nothing. He'd have got more raw speed out of a haircut.

Look at it this way. If you do the sums for the 2012 World Championships time trial course, a reasonably hilly 46km, you find that every kilo you saved in weight would gain something around six seconds. Every five watts you saved in aerodynamics gained about 16 seconds. For a serious bike rider on a serious bike, a kilo is a world of weight, and it has to be balanced against the consequent loss of power. Five watts, on the other hand, could be the difference between wearing sunglasses and putting a visor on your helmet. It's a few centimetres of exposed gear cable. It's nothing. There is probably no rider in the world who couldn't take five watts off his position or equipment for a time trial.

The other reason that aerodynamics has surpassed bike weight as a concern for professionals is that the UCI rules now impose a minimum weight on bikes. (The UCI rules, in all their strangeness and wonder, are something we will come back to shortly.) When the limit was originally set at 6.8kg it was very much at the lighter end of what was feasible. But that was in 2000. Today most of the mid-range bikes in your local shop are minimum weight. Pro bikes often as not have heavy components – steel pedal axles in place of the titanium of a few years ago, for example, or alloy bars rather than carbon – to make them heavy enough for the scrutineers.

Some minimum weight dodges are sneakier – the regs apply to track bikes too, which are even more likely to end up underweight due to the lack of brakes and gears. The trick used for a few years by one or two riders was to fill the seat tube of the bike with ice cubes, have it weighed, then park it somewhere warm (and perhaps over something absorbent) till the race. A small drain hole in the bottom of the frame was essential. A sloshing bike would arouse comment.

The starting point for any technical matter now is aerodynamics. After he retired from racing, Chris Boardman became the head of the GB squad's research and development team – known universally as the secret squirrels. He probably had more resources at his disposal than anyone else in the history of messing about with bikes. He didn't waste his time on insoles and ceramic bearings. As soon as he had a bike Sir Chris Hoy couldn't break, he did aerodynamics.

The more you find out about aerodynamics, the more difficult it all seems to get. It's still not all that long ago that the whole area was so utterly incomprehensible that there was not much point in worrying about it. You gave it your best guess and moved on. Once upon a time the cutting-edge way to optimise rider aerodynamics was by printing out photos of the rider taken head on, cutting them out, and weighing the paper. If you did this for a variety of positions on the bike, you found out which presented the smallest frontal area to the wind by finding the lightest bit of paper.

Things have moved on, and never once in the direction of simple. Just for starters, bikes go at just about the most awkward speed possible. Faster or slower would make life easier. Unfortunately, to explain why this is, you need to know what happens when air hits something – specifically what happens when it flows over it. The important bit is the boundary layer, the few millimetres above the surface of bike, wheel or rider.

Boundary layer air flows over an object in two ways. There is laminar flow, where the air flows in smooth parallel layers, and there is turbulent flow, where it tumbles and swirls. Both of them are attached to the surface – the air outside the boundary layer is unaffected, and flows round the object. (Nobel-prize-winning physicist Werner Heisenberg, he of the uncertainty principle, said that when he met God, he was going to ask, 'Why relativity? And why turbulence?' He said he believed God might be able to help him with the first one.)

A turbulent boundary layer produces a little more drag than a laminar one, so you'd imagine you'd want as much laminar flow as possible. But as the air flows over the surface, the depth of the laminar flow will increase, and then inevitably turn (trip) into turbulent. The later that happens, the more drag the turbulent flow will produce. That's the first issue. The second and more important is that a turbulent boundary layer will stay attached to the surface for longer. It will flow further round an object like a bike or a rider, leaving the air outside the boundary undisturbed, before it finally detaches, the thin boundary layer breaks down, and a large and hugely turbulent wake forms behind the object. The low air pressure of the wake will effectively 'suck' the rider back, so the less of it there is, the better.

The traditional illustration of this is a golf ball. A golf ball is actually not a bad model for a cyclist – it's a blunt shape for which aerodynamics is something of a secondary issue. A golf ball has dimples, because as the ball spins, the dimples trip the boundary layer into turbulent flow, which stays attached to the ball for a greater proportion of its circumference. Hence a smaller wake behind the ball, and smaller drag. A smooth golf ball would have a bigger wake, which would by yards outweigh the 'saving' of laminar rather than turbulent flow in the boundary layer.*

---

* The effectiveness of the golf ball's dimples has led several helmet manufacturers down the years to produce helmets with similar dimples on the front. The moment they find a rider whose head spins as they ride, they'll have the perfect headgear for him.

The problem with the speed bikes go at is that there is a lot of both laminar and turbulent flow going on. This means managing the transition from one to the other becomes a major headache. A Formula One car, for example, is in a lot of ways easier to deal with, because it's almost entirely a matter of turbulent flow.

So, armed with all this knowledge, what has cycling done with it? It's tempting to think we've done everything, just because we've done a lot. Bikes, wheels and handlebars have changed hugely over the last decade, not to mention the R&D methods used to develop them. But, like any other aspect of sports technology, it's a never-ending quest.

Boardman told me about a tour of the McLaren F1 factory-museum he'd been given by a senior engineer. When they got to the MP4/13 from 1998, the engineer said, 'When we did this one, we reckoned we were finished. It was perfect. It was the definitive F1 car. Two weeks later we had to put it back in the wind tunnel, and make it better.'

Formula One simply requires things to be improved on a continuing basis. Most of the aero work I've done over the past few seasons has been with another former Jaguar F1 engineer, Simon Smart, who told me that his department was simply told by the team management that over the course of the Grand Prix season they would improve the car's aerodynamics – specifically its downforce-to-drag ratio – by 10%. They had a graph on the wall with a line showing the rate of improvement that was required if they were all to continue to have jobs. If the line showing their progress that was drawn on top of it was higher, they were all happy. If it was lower, they were not. If they weren't finding more, they could be sure that someone else was.

In cycling, aero bikes hog the aero headlines. They look so fantastic that people with no thought of buying one still look at them longingly at bike shows. There is something glorious about the contradiction of a simple bicycle being designed to the very edge of what's technologically possible.

There are a few universals in aero bike design. Frames and handlebars have wing-profiles, with the aim of helping the flow to stay attached and preventing a wake. A wing-shaped 'tube' produces a tenth of the drag of a round one of the same frontal area. The details of the profiles and how the frame members join up are critical, but almost impossible to see, never mind to judge, by eye. At a more visible level the trends are towards integrated set ups. Smooth transitions from bar to stem to bike, all the cables hidden away, brake callipers built into forks.

In one or two cases, the attempts to manage the airflow appear more sophisticated. The time trial bike that Wiggins used at the 2012 Tour de France, for example, had a lip a few millimetres high zig-zagging along its down tube, presumably intended to trip the boundary layer from laminar to turbulent at an optimum point.

The attraction to an aerodynamic bike is clear – from the point of view of the rider, it's free speed. From the point of view of a team, if you get faster and better bikes, then the whole team gets the benefit. The development programme may be expensive, but unlike one-to-one coaching, it helps everyone. And at an elite level, the athletes are highly developed. Finding even a small improvement in a rider's engine might need months of work, altitude training, experiments with nutritional regimes, and might be derailed entirely by illness or injury. It might not even work at all, and even if it does, the gains will vanish much faster than they appeared as soon as the rider's form peaks.

If you make a bike faster, it stays faster, and it doesn't complain about the training load, being stuck at an altitude camp away from its family for weeks at a stretch, or having to drink a litre of beetroot juice every morning. Nor does it sign a contract with someone else at the end of the year because it wants more control of its image rights.

That's the upside. The downside is that the bike is a small part of the overall package. Take the wheels out of the equation, and a current top-level time trial bike accounts for about 300g of drag – which is only something around a tenth of the total. So, if we're dealing with a world-class rider, who can manage something like 470w for a long TT, the bike frame costs less than 50w. If you could make that 10% better, you'd have saved five watts, which would be nice, if not life-changing. The problem is that saving 10% on an already highly developed bit of equipment is exceptionally difficult. Much the same goes for wheels – they produce a little less drag than the rest of the bike. They've also been the subject of more R&D than any other bit of the aero jigsaw (small enough to fit in any wind tunnel, cheap enough to try anything with), so they're even more developed than bikes.

There are other complicating factors. The big one is yaw. Bikes usually get ridden outside, and outside there is usually wind. If there is any sort of crosswind, it combines with the forward motion of the bike to produce a 'headwind' that's off to one side – an angle of yaw. The best bike for a still day is not usually the best bike for a windy day. Most designers test bikes from zero up to 15 degrees of yaw – and the results can vary by most of half a kilometre an hour's worth.

More or less all the current aero bikes are actually faster in a crosswind than on a still day – the frame develops a small amount of aerodynamic lift that, while it doesn't push it forward, reduces the drag. This is why after decades of bike frames getting smaller and smaller and lighter and stiffer, with long seat pins and handlebar stems, bikes have been getting bigger again. The more frame there is, the more lift, the faster it ought to go. One or two recent world championship winners have looked as if they'd borrowed a bike from their big brother.

You have to design a bike with an eye to its likely conditions of use – a lot of triathlon bikes are designed in big yaw numbers because the Ironman Worlds in Hawaii is usually contested in windy conditions. You also have to bear in mind the speed of the rider, since slower riders experience greater yaw angles than fast due to the smaller proportion of their headwind that comes from forward motion. The fastest bike for a top pro might not be the fastest bike for a veteran amateur.

On the other hand, a useful side effect of yaw is that almost any bike will have a point in the wind range where it's ahead of all the rival manufacturers'. So everyone can put their hand on their heart and claim they make the most aerodynamic bike on the market. There will always be a day and a rider for whom they're telling the truth.

The bike designer's work is governed by a great many rules. The regulations governing what shape a bike can be for official competition are so involved and difficult to apply that almost no one understands them. I mean this literally – there have been several bikes designed by professional designers with the resources of very large bike companies behind them that were subsequently found to be illegal. That you might half expect, on the basis that rules are there to be diced with. What seems more peculiar is that in several cases the governing body (the UCI) initially decided bikes were within the rules, only to change their minds a year or two later, after a change of heart about what they'd meant when they created the rules.

Bikes have to be 'triangular', so they have to have tubes, or something like them. The frame members have to be of given minimum and maximum dimensions. They can't be more than three times as deep as they are wide, to prevent anything excessively wing-shaped. The dimensions of the tubes where they meet at the junctions between the frame members are tightly controlled. The rules are both complicated and vague, a combination that now means you have to give the UCI a sample of any bike you want to see used in competition for them to certify it as compliant. It seems not to have occurred to anyone that a set of rules so hard to understand that no one can be allowed to interpret them on their own might be fundamentally flawed.

Any sort of prototype or a bike custom-made for a particular rider is banned, and everything has to be commercially available – though quite what this means is not very clear. The Team GB track bikes and other equipment are available for purchase off a website for a price described only as being 'in line with the specialist nature of the equipment', and offering a lead-time that is simply 'long'.

These rules are a serious limit. One-piece frames like the Lotus are out, all sorts of experiments from the 1990s are out, all sorts of bikes from long before that are out too. My old Lotus hangs in my garage to this day, like the moon landings, a wonderfully advanced dead end.

I asked Simon Smart just how much of a limit the rules were. What could we do without them? What would we be riding now if the Lotus line had been allowed to continue? After all, the UCI rules only apply to UCI-sanctioned races – triathlon manages to struggle along with a rule book that says, pretty much, 'Is the thing in question a bicycle? Great, then get on with it.'

'We're looking at doing a non-UCI legal bike,' he said. 'But the problem is that people would have unrealistic expectations of how good it would be. The UCI legal bikes are very refined, we've worked on them for years, we've improved them again and again, and we know what we're doing with them. From a manufacturer's point of view, to start doing the same thing with non-UCI bikes might take five years of development.'

When I asked the same question of Boardman, he said that from his development point of view, the process behind the fastest legal bike was the same thing as the fastest bike. 'The rules make the whole things safer from a design point of view. You have to take fewer risks, because serious innovation is harder. Instead you can spend the budget looking for smaller margins.' The gains are in the details. Put it another way, the simpler you try to make it, the more expensive it all gets.

As an additional bulwark against originality, recent rules require any 'innovation' to be submitted to the UCI for approval before it can be used. The most significant invention of the last 30 years was probably the 'tuck' riding position that Graeme Obree devised, which was massively original, hugely effective, and required no more resources than turning the bars on a normal road bike upside down. The UCI had to go through a torturous and embarrassing series of rule revisions to get rid of it. That wouldn't be a problem now, because a new riding position could be banned before it had ever been used.

While the UCI bike rules are basically reactionary, there are some positives to be found. Boardman made the point that, structurally, the triangular frame shape they mandate is a great way to make a bike. That's why after decades of experimentation, it's the shape manufacturers always kept coming back to. It's telling that most of the Lotus bikes, overbuilt as they were, fell apart, because while the shape was aerodynamic, it was dreadful at coping with the stresses on a bike frame. They were made in left and right halves and bonded down the centre line, and eventually the halves would come unstuck.

This happened to mine during a race – the normal echoing rumble the hollow frame made was replaced by an odd buzzing. I noticed, with some alarm, that I could see the road surface flashing past not only on either side of the bike, but through the middle as well. I was about to hit the brakes, when I realised that if I did so, there was a good chance that the headset and front fork would just break loose and come backwards through the frame until the front wheel hit the back wheel, and I landed on my face. I freewheeled to a very ginger halt, and walked home. Sir Chris Hoy would have reduced a Lotus to carbon matchsticks.

Wind tunnel testing your riding-position is one of the most expensive ways of having a bad time yet devised. Each run takes several minutes, during which you have to maintain a position on the bike that is both perfectly consistent, and as still as is possible, given you also have to pedal. You can't move, because it upsets the measuring equipment. Rock a few millimetres back or forwards, or side to side, and the run has to be junked, and you start again.

You must accurately reproduce your normal riding position as a start point – even that isn't all that easy to do on an inanimate, bolted-down bike. Any new position you try has to be one you can ride in real-life – many riders have emerged from the tunnel with a new position only to discover they can't see where they're going.

(One or two of them, on mature reflection, have decided that seeing where they're going is a luxury they can do without. David Millar's late-period TT position meant that he was able to maintain eye contact with the team director in the car behind, or at least he could when his knees weren't in the way. He caught me once, and it was clear that if I hadn't got out of the way he'd have ridden straight over me. I don't think he'd even have noticed the bump – he was going so freakishly fast it was as if he was being pulled along by a magnet on a rail beneath the road.)

You have to do this without complaint as the warm 50kph wind sucks all the moisture from your body. A couple of hours in the tunnel leaves you like a heap of bleached bones on a tropical beach. All this for £500 an hour.

You do it because no matter how sophisticated your bike or wheels, the truth remains that you're seven times their size. Most of the drag comes from the rider, and just because the rider is a lump of meat and resentment, fashioned by evolution for every purpose other than aerodynamics, doesn't mean you don't have to make the best of it.

There are very few clear guidelines for setting a fast position. That's why you have to take yourself to the tunnel personally. What works for one body shape doesn't work for another. Is your back curved? If it's curved just right, the flow stays attached to it most of the way down to your backside. If it's curved just wrong, it detaches at the middle of your back, produces a wake like the Queen Mary, and leaves sparrows tumbling helplessly in your slipstream. Your back tends to be the shape it is. You're lucky, or you're unlucky.

The variables feel infinite – shoulder (or handlebar) height, reach, hand width, elbow width. Head high, or head low? Which helmet works with what head position? It's not just a case of 'bike-fit', moving the bars and saddle and so on. A great deal of what goes on in a wind tunnel has to do with how you sit on what you've got – do you scrunch your shoulders in? Normally that drops the frontal area a bit, which is good, unless it also pushes your head up, which is bad. Do you try to keep your back flat? That probably helps, unless it pushes out your shoulders again. Knees in? That depends, believe it or not, on what bike you're riding. After a few runs you start to feel like a poseable doll. With a sore neck.

Sometimes it's not even clear why something about a position works. I say sometimes, I mean almost all the time. I once asked Smart, after an especially confusing session, why putting my saddle forwards 20mm had produced a saving worth about 1kph. He told me that 'if' a position worked was a cheap question; you blew wind at it and saw what you got. 'Why' involved trying to work out what the airflow was actually doing. It was a very expensive question, albeit one which he would be delighted to help me with if I wanted to pay £500 an hour to find out.

The other thing you have to remember to do in the wind tunnel is to remember. If you discover that moving your elbows back 20mm, and shrugging your shoulders in a bit is significantly faster, you have to remember exactly how you did it, because the hole where 'why' should go means that you only know that that exact position works. You can't work it out again later, because you don't have the information.

During 2012, Wiggins invariably time trialled with his hands partially folded over each other on the bars. He had two 'B's tattooed on the backs of his hands (after his children, Ben and Bella) which aligned when they were in the right position. I've seen several people copy the hand position. I'm prepared to bet that the hand position itself matters almost not at all. I suspect it's simply a cue he uses to remind himself to do something else – perhaps it reminds him to get his head and shoulders in the right place. I can do something similar by squeezing the bars tightly for a few seconds every minute or two, which seems to pull my back into a shape that I know works.

If you're a time trial specialist, or a grand tour contender, all of this is something you have to take seriously. Exactly how much you can save varies from rider to rider, depending largely on how good a position they had to start with. In my case the numbers are confused by the amount of track testing – which I'll come to presently – I'd done before I went into a tunnel. A clearer example is British international time trial rider Julia Shaw, with whom I shared a sponsor, and consequently quite a few tunnel sessions. Julia was a national champion before ever seeing the tunnel, so was already using a position that was probably above average. Over the course of three or four seasons of refinement she saved most of 40 watts' worth of drag. For Julia, over a 40km time trial that's more than a minute and a half.

It's not impossible to find 40 watts by training, nutrition, and all the rest. But it's not easy, not at all. For a grown-up, experienced rider, it would be almost the difference between getting everything right and everything wrong, and most of us already like to think we're doing everything right.

Helmets were one of the first things the aerodynamicists turned their attention to, and one of the most visible. Conventional vented road helmets are an aerodynamic disaster – they're about a kilometre an hour slower than a shaved head or even a little cotton cap. But helmets designed for speed rather than ventilation are a different game. For a long time they were a real obsession, for many of the same reasons as wheels: they're cheap, easily interchangeable, and easy to test. There must have been a hundred variations on 'smooth at the front, pointed at the back', and with a few excursions into wilder, finned Flash Gordon numbers that were designed to appeal to those who wanted to look fast rather than go fast.

The oddest aero-helmet of the lot first surfaced as a computer-design file, released prior to the 2008 Olympics by the British team. It was extraordinary-looking – it covered most of the rider's face, and seemed to have barely an inch of surface that didn't have a fin, a duct or a vent to poke, prod or suck the airflow. Computer-generated arrows showed exactly how the air would behave – some going over, some round and some straight through the helmet.

It was a decoy. There was never any intention of making it. It existed exclusively so that news outlets would publish pictures of it. When the Olympics came round, the aero-helmets that the team actually used, while of a highly refined design, were fairly normal in their basic concept. I'd always assumed the red-herring helmet had been to encourage panic and unwise choices among the opposition. When I reminded Boardman about it, he said that anyone who knew anything would have known it wouldn't work. 'It was more about saying, "If we've tried this, can you imagine all the other things we must have tried? Just think how good the end result is going to be."' He also admitted that a consultant asked to produce 'the most aerodynamic helmet possible' had come back with an initial design that the rider couldn't see out of. You have to be careful how you brief.

The 2012 GB Olympic helmets were made of aluminium foam, rather than polystyrene. This made them smaller, which, if my knowledge of helmet aerodynamics counts for anything, would make them good in low yaw conditions, as you would experience on the track. Aluminium foam does not come cheap. You can buy the helmets from the same website as the GB track bikes and, as before, if you have to ask the price, you can't afford them.

While helmets have been an obsession for decades, skinsuits are an entirely new one. The stretchy Lycra suit has been around for decades. For most of those years everyone assumed that a stretchy suit was a stretchy suit. Anything that didn't flap was as good as it was going to get. Ideally it wouldn't have too many wrinkles either, but you can find plenty of photos of top level pros in the 1990s wearing suits that look like their mums had heard about the amount of human growth hormone in the pro peloton and wanted to leave space for a growth spurt.*

In 2002, the GB team developed a suit with dramatically reduced seams. There was one on the back of the shorts, one joining the shorts to the 'jersey', and some little tucks in front of the shoulders. Alwyn McMath, a team GB sprinter and my Northern Ireland Commonwealth Games teammate tried to convince me that one of these suits made more difference than an aero helmet, and I flatly refused to believe him. Instead I used a standard one provided by the team that was so big I resembled one of those cats that can turn round inside its skin and look out of its own arse.

When I finally laid my hands on one of the fast suits and did some track testing with it, I realised that Alwyn had been absolutely right. In the course of assessing equipment for an attack I made on the world hour record, it was one of the biggest improvements I found. Having switched to the new suit, it still didn't occur to me that there might be

---

* In the 1990s there were adult riders who went up a shoe size during the course of a season and gained hands like breadboards, while jawbone growth left large gaps between their teeth. You could spot them easily enough. They were the guys flossing with a dressing gown cord.

more to come from that line of enquiry. I hadn't twigged that skinsuits are a piece of technical equipment. Your skinsuit matters more than your bike.

Beijing 2008 saw a lot of clever stuff from Boardman and the squirrels. None was cleverer than the suits the track riders used. They were of a plastic finish, and weren't permeable by air. When combined with visored helmets and rubber overshoes that came halfway up the rider's calf, the only part of the rider that experienced any wind was their knees. The other peculiarity was that they were noisier to wear than fabric suits – the plasticised surface produced more wind-roar. It seems a good bet that increased turbulent flow was at least partly behind this.

They also had big, prominent seams. A strange development, after my experience with the older suit. The initial assumption was that this was simply how you had to join together the plastic suits. But there were other seams that were normal. It didn't take all that long to work out that the big ones were there for a reason. They were, of course, there to manage the airflow. They tripped the laminar flow into turbulent flow, at an exact point on the upper arms. Riders had lessons in how to put the suits on to get the seams in the right place.

There were also big seams on the chest, running diagonally from the armpits to the bottom of the sternum (called the xiphoid process, since you ask). While I had some, admittedly pretty erratic, success copying the arm seams by sticking duct tape edged with pinking shears over my normal skinsuit (and hoping no one started to wonder aloud just what the hell I was playing at), the chest ones never seemed to make any difference. I asked Boardman about this. He raised an eyebrow and said, 'You don't have tits, Michael.' I'd never noticed the final advantage to the suits' fabric. They could be made in three simple unisex sizes.

It's hard to judge exactly how good these suits were, since the testing data has stayed a secret. Clearly, though, the answer is somewhere between 'extremely' and 'unbelievably'. It was reported at the time that everyone who wore one set a new personal best. All the riders I've spoken to since who used one said that this was not an exaggeration. Estimates of savings were up towards three or four seconds over a 4,000m team pursuit – and when the riders are going at over 60kph, that margin is massive. It's far, far more than they ever saved by fiddling with bikes.

The plastic suits were banned not long after the Olympics. They were felt to confer an unfair advantage, and to unacceptably increase costs. British Cycling announced shortly afterwards that all the magic suits had been shredded, to prevent their secrets falling into the wrong hands. This was another nice piece of propaganda. The truth is they're still in a box somewhere in Manchester Velodrome.

Suits now have to be of a woven fabric – in practice the test is, 'can you blow through it?' And there is a stipulation that clothing may not be designed to improve performance via aerodynamics.* This is perhaps the jewel in the crown of daft UCI rules – there is almost no item of modern cycle clothing that is not, at least in some respect, designed with aerodynamics in mind. Otherwise we'd all ride in anoraks. No one would ever zip themselves into a tiny Lycra suit to ride a bike other than for the aero benefit. Nor would there be any other reason for anyone who wasn't certifiable to wear a helmet with a long point at the back, unless they were on their way to a pterodactyl-theme party.

---

* There is also a stipulation that clothing should not change the shape of the rider through compression. Clearly they heard about a former teammate who had himself wrapped around several times in gaffer tape to keep his shoulders in.

As is usual when a reactive rule is implemented to avoid costs and unfairness, it went wrong on both counts. The GB team response for the 2012 Olympics was to use the knowledge gained from the plastic suits to develop fabric suits. Plastic was simple – smooth is smooth. Fabric is harder, because the exact texture is critical. This, and the consequent drag, vary from one fabric to another.

They took samples of as many fabrics as they could find to the tunnel to test them. But it went beyond that. Boardman: 'I was sitting up in bed one night, going through some notes before going back to the wind tunnel in the morning. I mentioned to Sally [his wife] that we'd tested however many hundred samples it was, and just how absurd that was if you stopped to think about it. She said, "Did you test them wet?" I said that of course we hadn't, why would we? "You were always soaking when you got off a bike," she replied. And I thought, "Shit. She's right." So we went back and tested them wet. And the results weren't the same.'

He wouldn't tell me, but my guess would be that making the fabric wet made it smoother. In a world of fabric suits, the faster you go, the smoother you want the fabric. So a wet suit would be better suited to a faster event. I don't think they ever got to the point of different suits for differently sweaty riders. But maybe they will.

The suits they did use (and debuted by Wiggins a couple of weeks earlier at the Tour) continued the big seam theme, this time with lovely zig-zags that recalled my experiments with pinking shears and duct tape. The suits were bespoke for each athlete (unlike the plastic ones), tailored to each rider over three or four fittings. The rumours round Manchester Velodrome in the run-in to the Olympics were that these suits were actually better than the plastic ones – at a greater cost of development and manufacture.

As with the extensive rules about bike shapes, here the attempts of the rule makers to make things fairer and cheaper managed to achieve exactly the opposite. It's like tax laws. The more rules you have, the more loopholes you create, and no one with brains and funding ever looked at a loophole and decided to leave it for the next guy.

I'm worried that all this looks too easy. I wish that it were, but it isn't. Not long ago, I sat down and added up all the free speed I reckoned I'd gained over the last ten years or so. I had to guess some bits here and there, but overall I felt I had a decent grasp of the big leaps forwards. I have made four major position changes during that time, for example, and all of them were based on reasonably solid evidence. Skinsuits I've tested in the tunnel and on the road. Helmets, ditto, bikes, ditto, wheels, ditto. I didn't make any wild assumptions about how much I might have gained from one or two things I'd never really tested properly. I was realistic, perhaps even a little pessimistic. It was a nice, sober exercise to while away a quiet winter evening.

The problem was that when I added it all up, I should have gained about ten minutes over a 40km time trial. In reality I've probably gained more like two, maybe two and a half, and that's even after I've made allowance for the fact I don't have as much raw grunt as I did ten years ago. Something over seven minutes has escaped.

I don't know exactly where it went. Or, more accurately, I don't know exactly why I get the wild overestimate – however breathless I get about this stuff, I'm still aware that from a mental health perspective deciding that your model is right and reality is wrong constitutes a fairly big step. I should know better, but I still fall into the trap of assuming that, just because this is a part of cycling that deals with engineering and looks more controllable than the make-up of your muscle fibres, it's easy to predict what's going to happen accurately.

Everything interacts with everything else. A front wheel interacts with the forks, which both interact with the frame, and you interact with the whole shooting match. Even if all of that works, a gust of wind from the side will change how all the components work both on their own and together.

Try to imagine for a moment the complexities of the airflow round the top of a front wheel as it passes through the forks. While you're imagining it, remember that the wheel will be rotating – the top of a wheel is often moving at 100kph relative to the ground, and quite a bit of air will stick to it. If you don't believe me, get someone to hold your bike off the ground while they use the cranks to spin the wheel up to race speed. Put your hand close to the tyre – there is a lot of air being swept along. Consider that this hits the forks from one side and the wind generated by the bike's motion hits them from the other. Don't forget to allow for the brake blocks in there too. Same with the back wheel. Same with your legs and feet, and the cranks.

The more refined everything gets, and the smaller a gain we're prepared to try to nail down, the more troublesome it all is. A big improvement in, say, a front wheel would almost certainly translate into any bike frame. A small improvement may not – it may even be worse in a different set up.

When I was doing the interviews for this book, my conversation with Boardman took place in the stands above Manchester track a couple of months before the London Olympics. On the recording of the interview I can hear riders and coaches at an equipment-testing session in the background. My arrival in the track had caused some consternation. To get there I'd ignored lots of signs saying things like 'no entry' and 'no unauthorised personnel' that, it turned out, had been intended to include me.

'You didn't see any of this,' I was told, 'but you really, really didn't see those forks.' I could have quite honestly told them that up to that point I actually, actually hadn't even noticed them. However, when everyone started doing a sort of incoming-meteorite routine, I noticed that the space between the fork blades was huge – instead of tapering in from the hub towards the fork crown, they stayed dead vertical, and finished in a space above the wheel wide enough for a flat hand. They were subsequently used on the Olympic bikes. (But only when a front disc wheel was used. Wheels with spokes had a different fork design.)

What made this even more of an anorak magnet was that the 2008 bikes had used totally the opposite solution – really narrow forks that hugged the wheel and only flared out to the hub at the very bottom.

It's not hard to see how this happens – the first experiment was to make the forks narrower. That was better. Narrower still was better still. No one at that point tried the other solution, because obviously that would be worse. Except clearly it wasn't. The truth seems to be that, at least for the specific purposes of the GB track team, any solution is better than the conventional one.

'It's interesting,' said Boardman, 'all the first-generation wind-tunnel work we did translated really well into the real world. The results in the tunnel were the same as the results on the track.' First generation was the 2004 and (especially) 2008 Olympic cycles, when Boardman and several technicians contributed greatly to the world's sum total of completely normal things by moving into a wind tunnel in Southampton with a life-size, fully poseable model of Jason Queally and dressing it in a selection of plastic suits.

By the 2012 cycle, what they found was that things that looked good in the tunnel didn't work as well in real life. They came to use computer simulations more – known as computational fluid dynamics or CFD. All the key athletes were scanned into the software, along with all the bikes and equipment. Then ideas that looked promising in the CFD application were tested on the track with a power meter without going through a wind-tunnel stage at all.

The advantage of doing it this way is that you can leave the computer to get on with working its way through all the possible variations of position, equipment and clothing, and then see what looks promising. It avoids the danger inherent in a lot of marginal gains chasing, that of fine-tuning an idea that is basically wrong. Boardman didn't say so, but I'd be reasonably confident that the wide fork was the result of a computer burbling away to itself in the small hours of the morning, just trying anything that might fit within the possible parameters, uninfluenced by any preconceptions of what was supposed to work and what wasn't.

It's an odd echo of the early stages of Boardman's own aero career – testing the original Lotus he said that the most useful guy there knew nothing about bikes or cycling. 'He'd say, "Can you put your arms like this?" and the guy working with us who knew about bike riding would say, "You can't ask him to do that!" and we'd try it anyway, and see what we got.'

It was a theme of the conversation – that some of the big steps come from those outside cycling, or at any rate outside mainstream development. Graeme Obree, Sally Boardman and the wet suits, the Lotus testing, a computer that has the time and the patience to try anything, however daft. Looking to outsiders feels at odds with the culture of marginal gains, small improvements from detailed graft – except that marginal gains might not be the best way to describe what they're doing. It's not the gains that are small, or the approach to them that is small, but that where they go looking is small. It's not taking a whole bike and rider, or even a whole bike, and asking how to make it better, it's looking at every component, however trivial, and asking how that might be made better. Then checking again that the new, faster part is still faster when it's in the whole system of bike and rider. It's painstaking, and slow, and with every improvement you make, the gains that are left get exponentially smaller, but it means you look at things no one else has ever looked at.

It changes the culture, and it changes how athletes look at equipment. For a hundred years bars had been between 40 and 44cm wide. They just were. By summer 2012, the GB track sprinters were all on much narrower bars – the testing showed a small gain. A decade earlier, the riders would have found a reason to reject them: 'I can't breathe … I can't handle the bike properly …' Around that time I overheard the then head-coach Simon Jones asking a world-championship medallist to carry a power meter during a winter six-day track race, just to log data about how those events worked. He was turned down flat because, 'I'll look like an idiot, Simon. No one else is going to be using one.' In the current culture, riders had just said they wanted the gain, so they'd make the change.

The move to more CFD is interesting in itself. Wind tunnels have been the gold standard for many years, but even I've come across things that work in the tunnel, but don't seem to actually work in races. Oddly, the problem is not with the wind tunnels, but that we know far less about the real world than we ought. Tunnel tests run at angles of yaw, we know the effects, we can repeat the results consistently. What we don't know is what real angles of yaw riders encounter in the real world. One wheel manufacturer in a series of adverts some years ago claimed an average wind speed in the UK that was based on Met office data which is collected ten metres off the ground. There is a lot more wind up there than there is at wheel height. They'd spent hundreds of hours in the tunnel, but never stopped to ask about what was going on outside.

You can take a stab, clearly, and I've spent many happy hours standing by the roadside with an anemometer and a bit of wool on a stick, being mistaken for a simpleton. Even if it's all rather approximate, it's still more than most people are doing.

Another issue is our old friend turbulence. Smart pointed out that the wind in his tunnel was lovely and clean, all flowing nice and smoothly. As soon as you release wind into the wild, 'It blows through a hedge or round some trees or over a fence, it becomes turbulent,' he said. 'And that makes a difference.' Boardman might know more about it than he let on. A track is a more controlled environment, but even in a team pursuit on the track, the riders are in air disturbed by the other team. (TP squads are now getting so fast, around 14 seconds a lap, that in fact a team alone on the track is just about riding in its own slipstream.)

Smart told me that he's working on an answer, a probe for a bike that would measure real conditions: wind speed, yaw, turbulence. Initially an idea for helping to transfer tests out of the tunnel, he suggested that the next obvious use for such a thing would be for a rider starting early in a time trial to ride with the probe, to gather information to help later riders in the same team make more informed choices about equipment, clothing, even position. Personally I can't help thinking that if this project comes to fruition, the UCI will bite through the stem of its pipe in horror, but it's a fantastic idea.

Where it's all going next is no easier in this area than in any other. There are some refinements that aren't too difficult to spot – bikes are going to become more integrated, in that the wheels will be designed to match a particular frame, as will the bars and other items like chainsets. This will happen because a) it will look good, b) there'll be a few quid in it for the bike manufacturers, c) the pros will do it and d) it will be marginally faster.

Changing things like position for different conditions clearly has significant possibilities, but you need to know what the conditions are. You can't adjust your bike on the fly (rules, rules), but you can certainly change how you sit on it. For skinsuits with trip seams, it's probably possible to optimise where the seams go depending where the wind is coming from.

This chapter has been unashamedly concerned mainly with time trial and track technology – partly that's just a personal obsession, but it is also where you find the cutting edge of this stuff. It's where the rewards are clearest, and, at least as important, it's the area of cycling where riders have been forced to be receptive to change. But aero is taking over the rest of road cycling too. From the moment Mark Cavendish won the world championships in 2011 wearing a time trial skinsuit and a helmet with a plastic shrink-wrap cover, that's where it's been going.

It's a surprise that it's taken this long. At any speed above about 25kph, half the resistance on a bike is aerodynamics. By 30kph it's almost everything. Never mind the hero of the long break, even sitting in the shelter of the bunch, on the flat most of your problem is aerodynamics. Whatever energy you can save there, you can use somewhere else. Riders are taking road bikes to tunnels to do the same routines that used to be only for TT specialists.

There are compromises – a road aero helmet has less ventilation, a road skinsuit has to be a bit more comfortable if you're going to ride in it for hours, and it either needs pockets, or you need a teammate to carry the picnic hamper. Aero road bikes are already into a second and third generation. At the moment there is still a slight penalty for an aero bike, as it's still a case of picking two from light, aero and stiff. It won't be long till you can have all three, at least as long as you don't want cheap as well. Cheap has not happened in 160 years of bike racing. If anything it's getting further away.

The problem with all of this is that while it's all free speed, it's no use if everyone else has it too. In truth what I've been looking for all my life is free speed that only I have. That's what everyone else wants too. You can never stop looking for the next thing. I can't remember my partner's birthday, but I can remember every wheel, frame, handlebar, skinsuit and position I've ever tried, and what I learned from them.

Like everything else about bike racing, it's a process, not an outcome. There is never a solution, only the next step, one that in time will come to look comically wrong. The guys that do best are the ones who know how they're finding the next step, even if they don't know what it is yet.

CHAPTER 7

Talent and genetics

When I originally planned this book, I was going to include a slightly pretentious epilogue. It was going to consist of answers from all my interview subjects to the same, simple question, which was going to be, 'What makes a fast bike rider?'

In the end I came to think better of the idea, largely because almost no one gave me the straightforward one-sentence, one-thought answer that it relied on. To make it work would have needed too much editing and paraphrasing for it to ring true. It was probably just as well I gave it up. A neat series of simple answers – or worse, a neat series of the same simple answer – would have rather undermined the rest of the book.

It was worth asking everyone the question, though. If I had gone ahead and edited and paraphrased it, a pattern would have emerged. The riders almost all said that the answer was hard work. The coaches almost all said it was about a basic physical talent. One elite athlete turned elite coach even said that when he was an athlete he thought it was hard work, but now he was a coach he thought it was more complicated than that – it was clear to him now that the good ones were born with something.

The idea of a basic talent, something innate, something in the genes, is moderately controversial. Some elite athletes feel a bit insulted if you imply that at least some of how they got to where they are is indistinguishable from luck. Ambitious youngsters (and sometimes even more so their parents and coaches) don't like the idea that they're not starting with a blank piece of paper. That it's not all about hard work. That maybe you don't actually get what you deserve. Other athletes are intimidated for the opposite reason. They don't want to be told their body has all the natural talent in the world, and its failure to reach the pinnacle of the sport is all down to deficiencies of personality.

The idea of natural talent has taken a bit of a hammering in the last few years, in sport most notably from Matthew Syed in the book *Bounce*. The pleasingly simple essence of Syed's book is that it's all about practice. He buys into the suggestion of Malcolm Gladwell in *Outliers* that 10,000 hours of practice is a key factor in success in any field. Most probably that comes as ten years of 1,000 hours a year. That's what it takes to reach the top, and normally what looks like 'natural talent' can be explained by the fact that those who apparently have it also did a lot more practising as well.

Bounce is persuasive. It provides a convincing explanation for Syed's own Olympic table tennis career, the chess abilities of the Hungarian Polgar sisters, and the phenomenon of the child music prodigy. The book's limitation, and one that Syed is entirely upfront about, is that the examples it takes are almost exclusively ones that involve complex actions – golf, chess, table tennis, playing the violin.

Cycling is not a complex action. In terms of technique, the moment your dad lets go of you and you're wobbling along on your own, you've pretty much got the whole package. Everything from there on is just details. The only sport whose basic action is simpler is running.

When I took up cycling, I was good at it immediately. My second-ever ten-mile time trial, and the first one I did riding a time-trial specific bike, yielded a time of 19'44". That was one of the fastest times recorded in the UK that season. I won the race by over a minute, from riders who'd been training and competing for many seasons. My third ten-miler was good for about seventh in the British University Championships.

At my first ever open 25-mile race, I finished third, and the guy who finished fourth had to be physically restrained from attacking me at the HQ afterwards, so sure was he that I must have taken a shortcut. The guys restraining him broadly speaking agreed, they just didn't want to be responsible for explaining to the custodian of the village hall why there were bloodstains and bits of brain on his badminton court. Within a year I'd finished nineteenth at the national championships, in a field that included several pros and quite a few members of the GB Olympic team.

The margins by which I've improved since that first season have actually been quite small. I don't have precise data, because as a student I didn't have the foresight to blow my food budget for the next decade on a power meter. But in percentage terms, my best guess would be that my improvement since that first season was never more than about 15%, in raw power terms. I've no idea how that breaks down into the various aspects of physiology, but I would assume that most of it comes from greater efficiency. It would be fascinating to know exactly, but of course I never will.

There are objections to this. Even if we gloss over the anecdotal nature of the story, anyone who knew me at the time would simply have ascribed this sudden ability to ride a bike to a cross-over from another aerobic sport, that of rowing. The problem with that is that within about a fortnight of getting on a bike I was a better bike rider than I'd ever been a rower. That still applied even if you stripped out the technical aspects of rowing and just measured it on a rowing machine.

You could still argue that I couldn't say anything definitive till I'd done my 10,000 hours and seen what happened. Certainly I did keep improving over the next few seasons, but by the time my 10,000 hours arrived, I'd long since stopped making any significant progress.

The point, though, isn't really whether I got better or not. The point is about where I started out. The second-placed rider at my second race wasn't a pro, or even an elite amateur, but he was a rider with years of experience, and a lot of training and racing behind him. I still beat him by a margin greater than the improvements I made over the entirety of my subsequent career. To put that another way, he would have needed that ten years' worth of gains to get to the level where I began.

I'm quite convinced that I have a natural talent for bike riding. I have at least some natural talent for any aerobic exercise – I could win cross-country races at school for fun, but took care not to, so as not to have my Saturday mornings ruined by being required to turn out for inter-school competitions when I might otherwise be playing the bass recorder in the Belfast Early Music Society. I was a perfectly competent province-level junior swimmer too, despite a technique so random that it often took a skilled observer several seconds to decide if I was doing front crawl or back crawl or signalling for help. But when I got on a bike, something clicked. I could just do it, and even at the time I knew I had an ability I'd done nothing to deserve.

There are some athletes who agree with me, even if they're in a minority. Alex Dowsett mentioned a local rider we both knew, and said that he reckoned he trained harder and smarter than Dowsett had ever done, yet was no more than a good club standard. More than one person singled out the same senior road pro and suggested that if he'd ever done any serious training he'd have won everything there was to win from the Tour de France downwards. The problem was he was sufficiently talented to win quite a lot and earn quite a lot without the inconvenience of spending his days schlepping round the country on a pushbike, so he didn't bother. I remembered one conversation with the rider in question where I was genuinely amazed at the shambolic approach he had not just to training, but to being an athlete in general.

It was his choice – the same question of investment against potential return that everyone has to work out for themselves. If he was pushed towards doing more, he'd probably have quit the sport altogether in frustration and boredom. If almost anyone else in the pro peloton had been blessed with his genes, they'd have been the next Eddy Merckx. If I'd got them, of course, I'd have over-trained the hell out of them, but my second-ever bike race would have been even more of a showstopper.

That's the thing. I have a lot of talent. But there are plenty of people with more, even if some of them don't make the most of it. Equally, there are plenty of people with less natural ability, but who can still beat me because they worked harder and smarter and lived better. I can't help feeling they deserve their successes much more than I ever did. But that's introducing the ethics of a meritocracy into a world that I'm quite certain is a lot more complex.

In the 1980s I grew up in a world that seemed very enthusiastic about genetic determinism. I remember, just, a

BBC TV series called *Feeling Great!* It was a very basic fitness primer aimed at a generation that had just discovered jogging. I can recall little about the programme now, except that it advocated swimming as being best for the three 'S's: stamina, suppleness and strength. And it included an interview with Derek Griffiths who was both a children's TV presenter and a fan of cycling. He explained that one of the great things about riding a bike was, 'You can go out early in the morning in your vest and underpants, and there's no one around to say, "Look at that fool!"' I recall, even at a very tender age, reckoning there was a good chance he was wrong about that, an opinion that I am happy to stand by now.

There was a pamphlet to accompany the series, a copy of which ended up on the family bookshelf. It included a section on somatotyping, or body typing, accompanied by useful diagrams so you could identify your body type. You were a mesomorph, an ectomorph or an endomorph. A mesomorph looked like Zeus. An ectomorph looked like Michelangelo's David. An endomorph looked like a beanbag chair with a face and a bad haircut.

In a world of determinism, your shape determined your future. Zeus was not just handsome, he was strong, fit and swift. He was a charismatic leader of men. Other men wanted to be him, and women (who didn't seem to have somatotypes, they were just 'girls') wanted to be on his arm, basking in their good fortune. Ectomorphs were good at running. They were also neurotic, 'flighty' (whatever that means) and, if I recall correctly, prone to allergies. Endomorphs were 'easy-going', 'fun-loving', and were advised to limit their athletic activities to wearing a beer-hat and cheering on Zeus and David as they chucked spears and ran from Marathon with news of the victory.

I looked exactly like an endomorph. That is because I was nine, and almost all nine-year-olds look like endomorphs.

But I didn't know that at the time. The only hope for me was a footnote that said, 'You cannot change your somato-type, though there is some evidence that exercise during adolescence may have a small influence.' I was very lucky that I got there in time. My adolescence duly passed in a spasm of weightlifting. In the end I turned out somewhere between meso and ecto, but I'm sure that all that teenage clean and jerking had very little to do with it.

I was a little surprised to find that the idea of somatotyping is still around in academic literature, though it's used with a lot more caution these days. I probably shouldn't have been. While it's hard not to feel that judging people according to the ratio of their chest and waist measurements is somehow wrong, at a very basic level it's difficult to escape from the fact that elite marathon runners don't look a lot like Olympic weightlifters. Nor is it at all easy to persuade yourself that this is just a matter of training. They are, fundamentally, different shapes.

Cycling, at least, is a fairly accommodating sport. Anything on the meso-ectomorph spectrum seems to work perfectly well. Height isn't especially critical. Muscularity is a bit of a problem for road riders since it screws with their power-to-weight, but it's a necessity for a lot of track disciplines. You can't really spot a bike rider by simple shape. You need to look deeper.

The scientific basis of genetics is not intuitive. It's difficult, and often confusing. But a rough understanding of how it works does help make sense of how it affects sporting ability.

The double helix shape of DNA we all, probably, know about. The significance of it, perhaps not. The double helix is linked by a series of molecules, like the rungs of a spiralling ladder. There are only four of them − it's a bit like binary code, but in base four. The sequence of the rungs is the key. A sequence of molecules in the DNA indicates the order in which a series of amino acids are to be joined up to form a specific protein. A gene is the section of DNA that contains the instructions for a particular protein, and these proteins are what your body, its organs, its muscle, its blood, its brain, are made from.

The thing I struggle to grasp is the amount of genetic information your body contains. Not far from where I live in South Cambridgeshire, there is an unexpected union of cycling and genetics. Sustrans, the cycling charity, built its 10,000th mile of bike path from one of the local villages into Cambridge. To commemorate the significance of both the bike path and the deduction of the double helix by Crick and Watson just down the road in a pub in the centre of town, along the middle of the path is a barcode of 10,257 transverse red, yellow, green or blue lines. Each of the colours represents a molecule in the sequence of a gene. Each line is just a couple of centimetres wide. The path is over a mile long. That's just one gene, scaled up 750,000,000 times. The human genome contains about 22,000 genes in total.

The long strings of DNA containing all these genes are arranged on chromosomes, and the chromosomes form 22 pairs – one of each pair from each of your parents – plus either two X sex chromosomes (female) or an X and a Y (male).*

What creates genetic differences is not that you have a gene for 'x' or a gene for 'y', but that the genes have different variations. And it's these variations in the genes from individual to individual that create polymorphisms – differences in physical characteristics. Essentially 'having the genes to be a

---

* To be entirely accurate, the pairs of chromosomes are not quite 'one from each parent' – there is some cross over between them, so that while your genes are inherited, your chromosomes are actually unique to you.

cyclist' means a favourable combination of polymorphisms. The first genetic element that was isolated which was shown to have a substantial impact on sporting ability was the ACE gene (ACE stands for 'angiotensin I-converting enzyme', since you ask). It can come in two variants, either with or without an 'extra' 287-molecule sequence. The presence of the sequence is associated with higher VO_2 max, greater preponderance of type 1 muscle fibres, and an ability over long, endurance events, like road cycling. The absence of the sequence has an association with short distance power events, more like track sprinting.*

One study from 2008 set out to look at 23 polymorphisms known to be beneficial to endurance sport, and how frequently they occurred. Most of them were relatively rare. The researchers calculated the probability of any individual possessing all of them. So for the ACE gene, the probability was 21%. For the next gene on the list (ACTN3, which encodes a protein found in muscle fibres and has a role in determining muscle fibre type), the probability of the 'right' polymorphism was 18%. At this point, just two polymorphisms in, the cumulative probability of someone having both of them is 4%. When you keep on adding more sporting polymorphisms, you eventually find that the probability of the 'perfect' athlete, based on these 23 variances, is one in 1,212 trillion. There is a one in 200,000 chance that anyone in the world possesses the perfect set. Even if you settle for 21 of the 23, the odds for a single worldwide occurrence are only one in ten. In the UK, you might find a handful of people with 12 of the 23, but it's very unlikely you'd find anyone with 13.

---

* The ACE gene is a little unusual, in that either variation is advantageous to one sort of sport or the other. Most genetic polymorphisms are either 'good' or 'bad' for sporting ability, in a much more black and white manner.

There is also a very good chance that more than the 23 polymorphisms studied are actually involved. So you can add a few more zeroes across the board.

All that is before you start contemplating the odds of one of these rare flowers actually taking up the right sport, enjoying it, and being supported into building a career in it. No one knows just how many of these polymorphisms the current top athletes have, but it's almost certainly relatively small.

The question the study didn't answer is the one that most athletes would find themselves turning over in their minds in the small hours of the morning. Given just how gifted some riders clearly are, just how good would this one in 1,212 trillion athlete be? It's the kind of question guaranteed to keep you in a state of anxious wakefulness.

It's almost impossible to answer it in a meaningful way, because the quantitative contribution of each of the polymorphisms is as yet unknown. That didn't stop me asking one of the authors of the study, Dr Alun Williams of Manchester Metropolitan University.* 'They'd be off the scale,' he said. 'They would be unbelievably good.'

I asked if 'unbelievably good' would extend to my own personal nightmare, the athlete so gifted that they need never train, someone who could be a world beater after preparation not significantly more taxing than setting down their cigar and climbing aboard their bicycle?

'I would think so, yes,' said Williams. 'They probably couldn't get off with actually staying in bed all day, but I would think they could manage without specialist training.'

---

* It was an unusual interview, in that it concluded with Williams taking a blood sample from me for an on-going study into athlete genetics. I sent him an email the following day thanking him for his time, and saying, 'I hope the blood I gave you proves useful', which probably set off an alarm somewhere at the HQ of the World Anti-Doping Agency.

He told me about a study that took a group of rats, and tested their time to exhaustion running on a treadmill. The top 10% of performers were then bred, and the same with the bottom 10%. The progeny of each of those groups was subjected to the same protocol, and the top 10% of the top 10% was bred, and the bottom 10% of the bottom 10%. And so on. After six generations, the über-rats were between 150% and 200% ahead of the under-rats. After 18 generations, the divergence was more like 700%.* 'If you were in a position to do so, and were prepared to put ethics aside, you could achieve quite a lot with an athlete-breeding programme,' he added drily. 'The East Germans did make some moves in that direction.' The problem with that is that athletes take rather longer to reach competitive age than rats.

We will accept, for the moment, that athlete breeding isn't a realistic option, even if it could be a side-benefit of the GB system gathering all those horny young athletes together in Manchester, rather than leaving them scattered all over the country as those sports which have not yet got round to considering their campaigns for the 2036 Olympics do. Given that, and given the probabilities show that however wonderful they might be, the 'perfect' athlete is a practical impossibility, what is the real world influence of genetics on sporting performance? How much is you, and how much is your parents?

The best available answer to that seems to be from the Heritage Family Study – a long-term US-based public-health study that investigated variations in VO_2 max and its

---

* As Williams pointed out, there are limitations with time-to-exhaustion – namely that the speed of the test remains constant, so if you breed a rat whose thresholds have moved enough to put that speed the other side of a critical physiological parameter like OBLA, you can get a disproportionate improvement. There's not a lot of choice, though, since rats are not amenable to undertaking a voluntary time-trial protocol. Probably because they're too intelligent.

response to exercise across a large number of families.* It found that there was a much greater degree of variation between families than within families. The bottom line is that in practical terms both 'base' VO_2 max and its degree of responsiveness are about 50% inherited. So if you want a simple answer to the question, there it is.

VO_2 max is, as we know, not the be all and end all. Yes, if you take a large population and test for VO_2 max and endurance ability, there is a strong correlation. But if you take the top couple of per cent, the elite, and do the same thing, its effect is diluted by other factors like economy and sustainable-threshold levels. The problem is that VO_2 max is a key indicator of health status, so it's much easier to get funding for studies. No one seems to have done any really substantial work on the inheritability of most of the other variables.

On the other hand, we know that muscle-fibre type, which has a significant influence on a lot of them, is also about 50% inherited. Williams said he felt that the 50% figure was, for the moment, a pretty reasonable general reckoning for the influence of inheritance across most of the various factors involved in elite sport. He suggested that sprint ability might be a bit more, due to things like muscle mass and body shape, but there aren't actually any studies. But things keep coming back to the 50% idea.

It leaves you a bit unsure what to think. Clearly life is not a level-playing field. On the other hand, there's still a lot of space left to individuals to work hard and get somewhere. 'If you're straight-down-the-line average genetically,' I asked Williams, 'how good can you still be?

---

* 'Heritage' is a trying-too-hard acronym − it stands for HEalth, RIsk factors, exercise Training And GEnetics. Someone, somewhere back in 1992 when it started, must have been very pleased with that.

What happens if you train perfectly, eat right, rest and recover, and essentially nail the art of being an athlete?'

'You've pretty much described my rugby career,' he said. 'I knew what I was doing, I reckoned I was training correctly, doing things right, and certainly doing them better than several contemporaries who were still always faster. If you're average genetically, you can get to a very high level. But to get to the very, very top? Against people who work as hard and as intelligently, but have a better genetic baseline and a better response to training? You're not going to win.'

The baseline VO_2 max and the degree to which training will improve it are largely, but perhaps not totally, independent. Even if most genes are specific to one or the other, there are likely to be some that contribute to both. The degree of independence might go some way to explaining vanishing-junior syndrome – the phenomenally talented 15- or 16-year-old who slips away from the top of the results as they get older. Traditionally ascribed to girls and drink, it's at least as likely that they were lucky to have a good starting point, but unlucky not to have the ability to improve it very much. The average VO_2 improvement in the Heritage study was 19%. But some were as low as 5%, and some were up around 50%. The girls and drink are as likely to have been a comfort after the fall as the distraction precipitating it.

We're still a long way from the idea of genetic screening for talent. A 50% genetic contribution is a lot, but it leaves a lot of space for hard work; in a way both the coaches and the athletes are right. Even if the idea of screening itself became practical and was accepted ethically, picking two or three youngsters out of a school year, and deciding they're your team for the Olympics after next is not going to be effective, for the same reasons that non-genetic talent-search programmes have had such mixed success.

However genetically gifted you are, you still need to become an athlete, and to do the work.*

While the idea of genetic determinism is what tends to grab the imagination, the reality is that genetics is going to make a much bigger contribution to helping those who are already athletes improve than it is to finding the athletes in the first place.

At the moment, as we know, the basic modus operandi for an elite coach (or, for that matter, any decent coach) is to examine the demands of the event, examine the capabilities of the athlete, and set about making them match. Two young athletes with a similar profile will probably start off with broadly the same programme. Time, race results and training data will more than likely nudge their training in slightly different directions as it starts to become clear what works best for each of them. The more experience a coach has, and the more detailed the sports science support, the faster this learning process will be.

Genetics can be part of this. You might have two people who, despite a similar performance profile, actually respond very differently to training due to their individual collection of polymorphisms. 'You might have one athlete who responds exceptionally well to training designed to stimulate their cardiovascular system, but who responds poorly to work aimed at their muscular economy,' said Williams. 'So you'd have to emphasise the latter. You'd send them out for lots and lots of very long low-intensity rides to try to keep nudging the economy upwards. Then you'd introduce the cardiovascular work, the intensity, at

* For a broader overview of the roles that genetics can play in sport, ranging from aerobic ability to issues of motivation and commitment, see David Epstein's *The Sports Gene* (2013).

the very end, because you know you'll get an immediate, significant response to that. A sports physiologist will see that pattern now, but if you could back that up with a detailed knowledge of the athlete's genetics you could be much more confident about it.'

The logical extension of that is that you'd get a 19-year-old rider being told, with a degree of certainty, that if they wanted to win the Tour de France when they were 26, what they needed to do was spend five years putting a real emphasis on long, easy riding, before starting to go through the intensity gears when they were 24 or 25. Not only can you be more confident about it, you can make big decisions rather earlier in an athlete's career, which means a team can get more out of its investment, assuming it can tie its asset down to a long-term contract.

This is the area where genetics probably offers the most to sport – to optimising individuals, not to screening or managing large populations. The geneticist is going to be part of the athlete's support team, alongside the coach, the nutritionist, the psychologist and the rest. The details of the athlete's genetics are going to be another information stream going into the process.

Until quite recently, most of the interest in genetics has focused on the issues of polymorphism and heredity. That's not the whole story. Genetics is a bigger subject than that. The genes you're born with are just the start. They contain the blueprint for making proteins. The DNA sequence is transcribed into another closely related molecule called RNA. The double spiral of DNA unzips down the middle, and the RNA takes an impression of the rungs of the ladder. The RNA then scurries off, gathers up amino acids and joins them together in the order indicated, and the DNA zips itself up again.

But genes don't all generate proteins all the time. They switch on and off, and they often do so in response to a stimulus. This is what's known as gene expression. It's differences in gene expression that mean identical twins – who start off with exactly the same genome – are not exactly alike, and become increasingly different as they get older. It's because how they live affects what their genes do.

At a simple level it's possible to affect gene expression by diet – the reason omega-3 fatty acids in fish oils have an anti-inflammatory effect is because they turn down a gene that's responsible for creating inflammation. The targeted, sympathetic nature of the effect is why fish oil is a better means of reducing training-related inflammation than a more widely acting non-steroidal anti-inflammatory like ibuprofen.

Training influences gene expression by increasing the expression of genes responsible for things like building muscle mass. And gene expression also explains the effects and limitations of training. It's possible, indeed it's fairly easy, to change type 2x muscle fibres into type 2a, that is, to change the fastest-twitch fibres of all into slightly slower-twitch ones. Type 2x is only found in any large quantity in almost sedentary individuals – spinal chord injury patients, for example, or the bedbound. Almost any activity at all starts to turn it into type 2a.

But it is a great deal more difficult to change type 2 muscle fibres into type 1. That is, to turn fast-twitch muscle fibres into slow twitch-muscle fibres. There is some evidence that long-term, high-volume training may have this effect. But it's really not certain that it's possible, and even if it is, it's most definitely not easy. The proportions are a main determinant of sprint versus endurance ability and they are either fixed, or very close to fixed.

The reason for this is genetic. The genes for type 2x and type 2a fibres are on the same chromosome. Training moves what's known as a 'tag' from one gene to the other, turning off the type 2x gene and turning on the type 2a. The same process doesn't work for type 2a and type 1 simply because the gene for type 1 fibre is on an entirely different chromosome. This, finally, is an explanation for a phenomenon that sports scientists have known about for decades.

Fascinatingly, there is evidence that changes in gene expression may even be inherited, raising the possibility that what an athletic child inherits from an athletic parent may be more than just the polymorphisms, but some include benefit from their training history. The influence may even stretch back to several generations – so you can blame any sporting inadequacy on your parents for not only who they are, but what training they did and what they ate.

This sort of detailed knowledge of how training, diet and environment and even heredity can affect gene expression is at a very early stage. Like a lot of what else is happening in the area of genetics and sport, it's about people telling you what is going to happen next. Clearly, the more we know about these mechanisms, the more focused everything becomes, the less of an athlete's time and energy is wasted, and the better their performances (hopefully) become.

There is a legitimate fear that all this knowledge might not be used for entirely pure purposes. Cycling has, just once or twice over the last hundred years or so, run into areas of negotiable morality. Clearly it's almost impossible for anyone interested in sport to survey the exciting new selection of control-levers being made available by genetics and not wonder just what the dishonest possibilities might be.

Of course, no one who's really up to no good is going to be shouting about it. Williams agreed that, if you set ethics aside, there were almost certainly things that were within the area of current knowledge that would have significant effects. You can use an engineered virus to introduce new genes into organisms, and thus genetically engineer animals like rats for characteristics including increased muscle mass, lower body-fat, or reduced muscular fatigue, and several other things that would have a clear performance benefit in athletes.

There have been successful experiments using genetic engineering in mice and non-human primates to increase the expression of the gene responsible for EPO. These have included experiments that produced macaque monkeys with EPO expression that could be effectively turned on and off – 'like a tap', as Williams put it. 'One molecule introduced into the monkeys' systems would start the expression, another would stop it, and their haematocrit would go up and down accordingly.' The attraction of this possibility to the dishonest is, I trust, clear.

The risks of genetically engineering an athlete are, for the moment at least, enormous. They are far, far greater than the potential dangers from most pharmaceutical doping products, because most doping products are currently approved medications and the dangers come from misuse or incompetence. But even in current medicine, genetic therapies are a last resort – and they've generated a considerable amount of collateral damage along the way due to unexpected side effects.

In one macaque EPO experiment, for example, the monkeys' red-cell count went up as expected, to the extent that in order to avoid the sludge-like blood causing heart failure, quantities of it had to be removed to allow plasma to thin out the remainder. But then a little further down the line several of them developed an entirely unexpected and very severe anaemia. The conclusion was that an immune response of the monkeys had produced antibodies against EPO that worked to neutralise not only the 'new' EPO, but the monkeys' own endogenous EPO, halting all red-cell production. The experiment had introduced a new autoimmune disease.

What happens when gene therapies are more reliable might be another issue. To take it to a distant extreme, how would sport deal with the situation where a normal, safe, reliable genetic modification was used by a large proportion of the population to make really substantial improvements to their health – say by reducing body-fat levels, or increasing muscle mass? At the moment, most doping legislation is pinned on the idea of risks to health as a justification. Where it's not, it often relies on at least a large degree of artificiality. But, to pick one example, caffeine has a substantially greater performance-enhancing effect than numerous banned substances. But it isn't banned because it's a normal part of life, and because the health risks are not all that great.

It's not hard to imagine genetic therapies with much more profound effects, but similarly low risk and 'weirdness' factors, becoming almost as common as a coffee habit. Williams had a pleasingly dystopian view of a world where genetic modification was common, but where it remained banned in sport. 'You could end up with a world where athletes are the weakest, slowest and least healthy members of society.'

Gene doping is not easy to detect, at least not at the moment. Biological-passport-type programmes that included the right parameters are probably the way to do it, where you look for unexpected variations. The macaque monkey EPO experiment wouldn't go undetected for long in even a current-day athlete.

It is, like everything else surrounding genetics, a work in progress. A common theme among sports scientists seems to be the idea that everything is turning out to be genetics – one of them said simply that 'all biology is genetics' – and he seemed to say it with the gloom of someone who felt he'd done the wrong PhD.

At the moment the details of how genetics is going to work in sport, and how sport is going to respond, really aren't all that clear. The amount of information that's waiting to be unlocked is vast. The uses to which it could be put vary from making marginal improvements to current talent identification programmes and training methods (pretty much a certainty) to bringing the whole edifice of sport crashing down (highly unlikely). For an athlete the whole area feels intimidating, because it seems so far beyond an individual's control. But that doesn't make it so very different from many other elements of sports science. The chances are that in ten or 15 years time it will be settling down into just another part of how elite performance works.

AFTERWORD

The never-ending search

I'M AWARE THAT I MAY HAVE MANAGED TO MAKE THE ART OF fast bike riding look awfully complicated. The problem is that going quickly, really quickly, is quite involved. At the top level, cycling is about keeping on top of the details. Looking for the margins and the tiny gains is what drew me into the sport, and it's still what I love about being a bike rider.

It's not exclusively personal. Like any other fan I adore watching racing in the high mountains, riders attacking, falling back, suffering and hanging on before finally, maybe, raising the energy to attack again. Or, on the track, seeing powerhouse riders leaping from almost stationary to 70kph in just a few turns of the pedals. The thing is, I adore it even more when I know what's going on, what's happening to them, why exactly they can do what they do.

I will try to untangle a few basics. For a moment, let's zoom out to the picture that includes all of us, from once-a-week cafe riders to Olympic gold medallists. In wide-angle, it's quite simple. For endurance riders, almost the whole difference between one end of the bell curve and the other is the ability to move oxygen. In practice, that's about moving blood. For sprint riders, it's about bigger muscles with the right mix of fibre type.

That's the most elementary possible set of answers, and if you want to know why Chris Froome is faster than Boris Johnson, that's why. If you haven't got those basic characteristics, you're not a fast bike rider.

The only reason it doesn't end right there is something you can find in simple studies that correlate VO_2 max and cycling ability. When you include a large, randomly selected population in a study, the relationship between VO_2 max and power output is a simple, very clear linear one. The bigger the VO_2 max, the faster you can go. For a large sample, VO_2 max is an outstanding predictor of cycling performance. But when you take just the top 2% of the sample and repeat the analysis, the correlation between VO_2 max and power is a great deal less strong. In a small sample of similarly able athletes, the variances created by everything else that's going on start to become as significant as the shifting of oxygen.

I share that final segment of the bell curve with Wiggins, Froome and the like, and the difference between them and me isn't oxygen shifting – I'm as good at that as any of them if not better – it's using that oxygen efficiently when it gets to the muscle. In other words, the difference between a fast rider and a slow rider is not necessarily the same as the difference between a very fast rider and a very, very fast one.

The closer you get to the top limits of performance, the more important the details get. Elite riders can't make much progress by simply training 'more' as they're already committing all the resources their bodies have. They, and their teams, are prepared to accept smaller and smaller improvements as being worth the effort. I've laid out the result of that detailed approach – the sheer number of tiny gains that are sought out, one by one, and piled together to find just a few seconds in a time trial, or the width of a tyre in a sprint. That's why it seems complicated.

In some ways, though, 'marginal gains' is a very swishy term for a fine-print pursuit of the moderately obvious. Almost every advance it produces is something you feel you could have worked out for yourself if you'd had the time and the money. As practised by the British track programme and the more determined pro teams it's been evolution conducted at a break-neck pace, but it hasn't been a revolution.

I don't for a second mean that in a negative way. If it was that easy to expend time and money efficiently, we'd all be doing it. Neither would I want to skip over the sheer balls required to look at something that has been done the same way for decades, and decide that it would be better if it was done your way. ('We've never done it like that' has changed its significance from a 'no' to a 'we'd better try it'.) 'Marginal gains' culture tends not to produce something that leaves you gasping in admiration of an intuitive leap. It's more likely to leave you overawed by the fineness with which it sifts its way through all of cycling looking for nuggets of speed.

As often as not what the top teams have done over the last few years is work through best practice from several other relevant sports: specificity in training from swimming, rowing and athletics, the idea of faster clothing from sports like swimming, and better aerodynamics and bike-technology from motorsport. As the next few seasons pass, it's going to take more and more originality and imagination to keep finding an edge.

Even things that will make a difference, like the better use of genetics in training – are going to tune in gradually. There is a good chance that most of them are going to be based on published research, which dramatically reduces the length of time for which one team or individual can have an advantage to themselves.

The positive to the arms race in cycling at the moment is the degree of openness. It's hard to keep bike technology secret when you have to ride it in public, and it's hard to keep training and recovery techniques secret when riders can come and go from team to team. There's no omertà surrounding interval sessions. For a certain sort of slightly geeky cyclist or cycling fan, it's an added dimension to the sport.

I occasionally wonder whether the diminishing returns from the scientific approach are going to push doping forward again as a temptation. It's possible to get a legal advantage at the moment if your coaches and sports scientists are ahead of the game. When the playing field starts to flatten out again, maybe more new riders will go looking for old advantages. At the moment, blood manipulation is still the most important part of doping, but it's getting harder to conceal. Different methods that are harder to spot might prove too much of a temptation.

Right now it's not really very clear what gene doping might have to offer, or the extent of the risks, or how easy it's going to be to detect. But it's quite certain that someone, somewhere will want to find out. That's when we'll discover whether the recent shifts in cycling's approach are based on an outbreak of genuine honesty, or were just motivated by better testing.

What it takes to succeed in cycling hasn't changed. The best riders are half-born, half-made. In other words, they're made up of a combination of talent and commitment. That has applied, and will apply, to everyone who ever made it to the top, from the first bike racer to the last.

How to succeed has changed, a little. The life of a pro bike rider has become more sophisticated. You don't have to go back too far to find that a pro with a coach (as opposed to a doctor) was a rarity and training was almost entirely homogeneous. It was just huge off-season mileages, plus days and days of racing. A lot of pros might have thrown something random into the mix – in the early 1980s British rider Sean Yates was notorious for a press-up habit that gave him the biggest shoulders in the pro peloton until the team management stopped him. But it was all sledgehammer stuff, and only the toughest could survive, never mind thrive.

Better training is much more closely tailored to individuals. Riders can succeed now who once would have been battered to their knees. In that respect it's easier for a rider to reach their potential – fewer genuinely talented, hard-working riders get wasted.

The downside is that it's harder now than it ever was for a maverick one-off of a rider to suddenly blast their way to the top because by sheer hazard they happened to stumble on a training method or a riding position that, for them at least, was phenomenally effective. There have been a few of them down the years – the most notable probably being hour-record holder Graeme Obree, whose success was based on two different but equally off-beat aerodynamic positions. His heyday was in the mid-1990s, when the universal reaction of the cycling establishment was to laugh at him, even as he demolished world records, because everyone knew that you didn't ride a bike like that. Almost no one seriously set out to investigate the potential of his approach.

He would find life much harder today. Even setting aside the rule-changes that effectively ban anything other than the most incremental innovations in equipment, the attitude from the rest of the bike-riding world would be more inquisitive. No one who was serious about it would dismiss something on the basis that it didn't look right. The first generation of aero road-helmets that left David Millar so closely resembling a man with half a watermelon on his head was a case in point.

The sport is more collaborative. Never mind being an outright maverick, it's harder than ever to get near the top on your own even by monotonous, grinding diligence. There's too much you need to be on top of. My own career path would be almost impossible today, because starting out on my own in my mid-twenties I would never attract the attention of the sort of people who could give me the help I'd now need. Thirteen years ago I could give my time trial position a best guess based on a few photos of Lance Armstrong, and since everyone else who wasn't the actual Lance Armstrong was doing the same thing, I wouldn't be giving much away. Now, I'd be surrendering more than I would ever get back by just kicking the pedals round.

You can buy the help, obviously. But no one who was an indigent proto-pro would be able to afford it. More than ever, even if you have the talent, you need the support of a team, and the way to do that is to get picked up early, at an age when you've clearly got quite a lot of bike riding left in you.

At least, that's the case for men. Historically, the smaller numbers of women competing in cycling makes it a little easier to come to the fore later. The shamefully small amounts of money available in women's cycling also mean that, for the moment at least, it lacks the investment that in men's cycling quickly puts major distance between those who made it on to the team bus as juniors and those who didn't. (It's worth saying, though, that this is beginning to change in some areas, most obviously national track teams.)

Is there anything I wish I'd known ten years ago? Of course there is. There's pretty much a book-full of it. Not just about how to approach the task, but the details as well. I'd have taken nutrition a lot more seriously. I reckoned that as long as I wasn't too hungry and wasn't too fat then things must be in a rough equilibrium, and I couldn't be doing that much wrong. In truth, I think I was giving a lot away for nothing. I could have gone faster for no more time or money, just a little more attention to detail.

I'd have trained with more specificity. I'd have tried to look at the demands of my events more closely, rather than just train hard and race hard and hope for the best. I'd have done what I do now, and spent a lot more time riding in my low-profile race position and a lot less on a normal, more upright road bike. And I'd have backed away from the long, long training rides that I did in imitation of the big stars, whose ability to recover from the depths of exhaustion turned out not to be based on their careful selection of vegetable juices. All of that would have made me quicker, and it would have been perfectly possible to have done things that way.

It would also, I suppose, have been useful to have known some of the details that have come about from research that's only been done in the last few years, but that wouldn't be so much hindsight as time travel. If I'd cracked that, I'd be a very fast bike rider indeed.

It might have been nice to do some things differently, but I don't plan to lose much sleep over it. The thing that I keep thinking about is how lucky I've been to have had some basic talent, and to have discovered a sport that it fitted so well. I was lucky that I walked out of a terrible job with no contingency plan, and stumbled into a series of sponsors who were prepared to pay me to chase a personal obsession. Finally, I was lucky that even after I retired from full-time riding I ended up doing a job that practically encouraged me to keep pursuing what I loved.

The whole art of fast bike riding is a process. The pleasure of it is not so much in the end result, but in the experiments and the discoveries. I like knowing that since the first bicycle there have been people like me, who wanted nothing more than to ride better, and I like knowing that there will never be an end to the search. Someone somewhere will always be working on a way to go faster.

Acknowledgements

This list of names seems a very slight recompense to all the people who helped me with the research for this book. All I can say is that I am hugely grateful to all of them. Not only was everyone I spoke to generous with their time, they were generous with their knowledge of elite cycling and cyclists, and our conversations were invariably both an education and a pleasure.

A great deal of help came from staff of Team GB and Team Sky, both based at Manchester Velodrome: Sir Dave Brailsford, Sir Chris Hoy, Dame Sarah Storey, Barney Storey, Chris Boardman, Dr Steve Peters, Shane Sutton, Dan Hunt, Paul Manning, Nigel Mitchell, Rod Ellingworth, Fiona McCann, and Abby Burton all very kindly took time off from the business of winning the world's biggest bike races to help me.

Emma Pooley, Alex Dowsett and Mathew Hayman provided valuable insights from their own experiences of riding at the highest level.

At Manchester Metropolitan University, Dr Alun Williams did an excellent job of making the genetics of sport comprehensible to a layman. He was also kind enough to read and comment on an early draft of chapter seven. At Smart Aero Technology, Simon Smart was patient in his explanations of the considerable complexities of cycling aerodynamics.

My own coach, Dr Jamie Pringle, has provided not only coaching over the last decade, but an introduction to the world of exercise physiology and sports science. It would not be an exaggeration to say that I wouldn't have written this book without him.

At Bloomsbury, I'm grateful to Charlotte Atyeo for the editorial whip-cracking, and to Jane Lawes and Ellen Williams. At David Godwin Associates, I'm indebted to Anna Watkins, and to David and Heather Godwin. Oliver Roberts (a man who is usefully both a coach and an editor) read a draft of the manuscript, and made numerous helpful suggestions in the cause of both accuracy and clarity.

Finally, my thanks to my partner Louisa for her patience through the years of obsessively pursuing the goal of faster, and then through the process of writing about it.

Index